DATE DUE

Library Store   Peel Off Pressure Sensitive

Medicolegal Investigation

of

Gunshot Wounds

Medicolegal Investigation
of
Gunshot Wounds

Abdullah Fatteh

M.B., Ph.D., LL.B., D.M.J. (Clin.), D.M.J.
(Path.), M.R.C. Path., F.C.L.M.

Deputy Medical Examiner, Broward County,
Florida; Visiting Professor of Pathology, College of
Medicine, Medical University of South Carolina;
Consultant, Criminal Justice Institute, Fort Lauder-
dale, Florida.
Former Professor of Pathology, East Carolina Uni-
versity, Greenville, N.C.; Associate Chief Medical
Examiner, State of North Carolina and Associate Pro-
fessor of Pathology, University of North Carolina,
Chapel Hill, N.C.

J. B. LIPPINCOTT COMPANY
PHILADELPHIA • TORONTO

In thankfulness dedicated to
my wife
MAHLAQUA
and to my children
SABIHA, FAIZ *and* NAAZ

ISBN 0-397-50356-3

Library of Congress Catalog Card Number 76-6957

Printed in the United States of America

6   5   4   3   2   1

Library of Congress Cataloging in Publication Data

Fatteh, Abdullah.
  Medicolegal investigation of gunshot wounds.

  Bibliography: p.
  Includes index.
  1. Gunshot wounds.   2. Forensic pathology.   3. Forensic ballistics.   I. Title.
  RA1121.F3   614'.19   76-6957
  ISBN 0-397-50356-3

Foreword

The investigation of gunpowder and perfection of the firearm are two of man's most significant achievements. The ability to cause and control a sudden release of energy and to direct that energy in a specific direction with reasonable accuracy have enabled him to explore, develop, and control vast areas of the world. The use of firearms has been a source of power as well as a means of pleasure and accomplishment. It has also been a cause of grief and sorrow. The firearm is but an extension of the good and the evil in its user.

The firearm reached its highest form of development, in one sense, as a military weapon. It is in that context that it has also plunged to some of its deepest depths of depredation. The firearm, in much of the world, also enjoys widespread civilian use. The United States is perhaps unique in legislating a constitutional right of the people to keep and bear arms. Unfortunately, throughout our history, there has always been a segment of our society that uses its firearms in an unlawful or antisocial manner. There will be continuing debate concerning the guidelines that our society can draw in an attempt to discourage the unlawful and improper use of firearms. The debate may never be resolved to the satisfaction of everyone. But whatever may come of attempts to lawfully regulate firearms in the United States, it can be predicted with assurance that there will continue to be injuries and fatalities due to the accidental, ill-advised, intentional, or unlawful discharge of firearms.

There is little likelihood that the number of firearm injuries and fatalities in this country will be materially reduced in the foreseeable future in our civilian community. The epidemic will continue. Those concerned with treating its victims should inform themselves of the characteristics and the interpretation of its lesions so that they may properly interpret these firearm injuries. Physicians and surgeons who examine the wounds in order to treat the living or to pronounce death should know the cardinal features of the interpretation of gunshot

v

wounds, since their characterization of the wounds may be the only record available for other investigators and the legal process. The law enforcement officer and the criminalist likewise need to recognize the different forms of wounds so that they may rapidly evaluate the case and plan their course of action, and be able to confer intelligently with the physicians and the lawyers concerned with the case. Attorneys, particularly those involved in criminal trial practice, also need to know about firearm injuries and fatalities in order that they may properly serve their client, whether it be the State or the defendant. And the judges, who may have ultimate responsibility for the evaluation of a disputed gunshot situation, should understand basic firearm wounding patterns so that they may properly evaluate the evidence adduced in court and assure themselves that a jury does not grossly misinterpret the medical evidence. Finally, the interested citizen who may want to learn something about firearm fatalities should have available a resource work that he can consult when public debate over firearm fatalities and the opinions of the medical and other experts erupts onto the front pages of the daily newspaper.

Everyone with an interest in firearms and the interpretation of firearm injuries and wounds upon the human body will benefit from Dr. Fatteh's work. Competence and confidence in the medicolegal interpretation of firearm wounds is essential to the proper administration of justice in our society today and in the future.

DAVID K. WIECKING, M.D., LL.B.
Chief Medical Examiner
Commonwealth of Virginia
Professor of Legal Medicine
Medical College of Virginia
Virginia Commonwealth University
Richmond, Virginia

Foreword

The past three decades have seen a rather dramatic change in the United States in the conduct of investigations into deaths subject to public inquiry. In many jurisdictions the outmoded coroner's system has given way to the modern medical examiner's investigative systems, many staffed by trained forensic personnel. It is a fact however, and will continue to be so, that a good proportion of medicolegal inquiries must be made by physicians who are not full-time forensic practitioners. To provide competency and to keep them abreast of the latest advances in the field, authoritative textbooks that will provide much of the expertise that they will need in a given situation are required. There are a number of excellent general textbooks in the field available, but there is a dearth of monographs devoted to a single subject. Since gunshots contribute so markedly to violent deaths in this country, a volume devoted to this subject is most timely.

Dr. Abdullah Fatteh, a prolific contributor to the forensic literature and an acknowledged expert in the field, has authored an important contribution to forensic medicine. Beginning with an excellent account of the historical aspects of firearms, he deals with every conceivable aspect of gunshot wounds. Even to the everyday practitioners of forensic pathology with much experience, the identification of entrance and exit wounds in many cases can be extremely difficult. Although the expert will find this work useful, to the physician who engages in the occasional practice of forensic pathology it is a godsend. Indeed, all of those associated with firearm injuries, from the police investigator to members of the bar, will profit from the content of this work.

GEOFFREY T. MANN, M.D., LL.B., F.R.C. Path

vii

Preface

In our society the gun is a constant threat to our safety, and indeed a common killer. Gun-related injuries are one of the leading causes of death in most of the United States. Abundance of guns makes the United States the most heavily armed nation in the world: there are an estimated 40 million handguns in the hands of the Americans, possessed either legally or illegally and 2½ million more are sold every year. These handguns and other firearms kill approximately 25,000 persons each year. The guns are very much a part of the American crime scene. For instance, 67 per cent of all murders in 1973 were committed with guns, the handgun being responsible for 53 per cent of the murders. A handgun is sold every 13 seconds and it takes one life every 48 minutes.

This high death rate from firearm injuries is not helped by the gun laws; present gun laws in the United States are both inadequate and unsafe. In 42 of the states no license is required to possess a gun, and in 30 states there is no waiting period for its purchase. Thus, guns are too easily available, too easily bought, and hence too easily used.

The high rate of injuries and deaths caused by guns involves almost every law enforcement agent, medical examiner or coroner, and attorney in the investigation of these injuries and deaths. This, therefore, is a compelling reason for writing this book, especially because no work dealing with various practical aspects of medicolegal investigation of firearm injuries and deaths is available at the present time.

The principal considerations in the book are the investigation of the scene of death or injury, collection of evidence, procedures in the autopsy room, follow-up investigations and documentation of the results of investigations.

The success of an investigation depends on the understanding of the precise role of an agency and the degree of cooperation among various investigating groups. An attempt is made in this book to delineate the duties and responsibilities of the police investigators and the medical men. The law enforcement agents, therefore, will discover clear guidance on how to approach a case of firearm injury or death. For the pathologist, the methods of documenting various findings on appropriate charts and diagrams are described. These investigators will also find helpful information about some of the newer techniques that can be used in the investigation.

A criminal lawyer probably prosecutes or defends more cases of firearm homicides than any other type. He will gain quick insight into the methods of investigation of firearm deaths and appreciate the extent and limitations of such investigations.

It is hoped that anyone involved in the investigation of the cases of firearm injuries or deaths, be he a police officer, a medical examiner, a coroner, a pathologist, or an attorney, will find this work useful.

ABDULLAH FATTEH, M.B., Ph.D., LL.B.

Acknowledgements

I wish to express my deep gratitude to many friends and colleagues who gave so generously of their time. My special thanks go to Dr. Geoffrey T. Mann, Medical Examiner, Broward County, Florida and to Dr. David K. Wiecking, Chief Medical Examiner, Commonwealth of Virginia. They reviewed most of the chapters for scientific accuracy and made many valuable suggestions. The chapters on Modern Firearms and Forensic Ballistics were critically reviewed by Dennis Gray, Firearms Examiner, Broward County Sheriff's Office Crime Laboratory and the one on Current Research in the Investigation of Shooting Cases was reviewed by Walter Matusiak, Toxicologist, Office of the District Medical Examiner, Broward County. I am grateful for their assistance.

I am indebted to Dr. Page Hudson, Chief Medical Examiner, State of North Carolina for the opportunity to consult and use valuable records and photographs in his office. The forms used in the text were originated by Dr. Geoffrey T. Mann when he was Chief Medical Examiner of the Commonwealth of Virginia.

I am thankful to Dr. Thomas T. Noguchi, Chief Medical Examiner-Coroner, Los Angeles County and Appleton-Century-Crofts for permission to reproduce parts of the autopsy report on Senator Robert F. Kennedy in Chapter 16 (From Noguchi. In Wecht, Legal Medicine Annual 1973. Courtesy of Appleton-Century-Crofts, Publishing Division of Prentice-Hall, Inc., Englewood Cliffs, N.J.). Appleton-Century-Crofts were also kind enough to let me use the text dealing with epidemiology of shooting deaths in Chapter 11 (From Fatteh and Hayes. In Wecht, Legal Medicine Annual 1974. Courtesy of Appleton-Century-Crofts, Publishing Division of Prentice-Hall, Inc., New York.).

Several individuals have helped, in one way or another, in the preparation of this book. I am especially grateful to Dr. J. E. Embry, Det. Sgt. Joseph Marhan, Det. Sgt. Richard Simpson, James Bailey, Thomas Thuma, William Brinkhous, and Lou Toman.

I thank Jo Ann Bell, Director, Health Affairs Library at the East

Carolina University, Greenville, North Carolina for her assistance in tracing and checking references.

The arduous task of typing the manuscript was in the capable hands of Judy Bok, to whom I am indebted for her care and patience.

Finally, it is a pleasure to acknowledge the cooperation of the staff of the J. B. Lippincott Company. To George F. Stickley, Vice President and Editor, Medical Books; Carole F. Baker, Copy Editor, Medical Books; J. Stuart Freeman, Jr., Senior Editor, Medical Books; and Fred Zeller, Vice President, Marketing, Medical Books Division, my special thanks are due.

Contents

1

Historical Aspects of Firearms

Man, being weaker than many animals, sought to create in ancient times a means of defense. The gun is the outcome of these endeavors. To fight offending forces from a distance, man in ancient times used stones, spears and slings. Then came the era of bow and arrow and the crossbow. The invention of gunpowder and the use of guns followed.

GUNPOWDER

The invention of gunpowder had to precede the development of guns. A considerable amount of literature, full of controversy, exists about the origin of gunpowder. According to Professor J. K. Partington, a British chemist, the Chinese knew about and used saltpeter-based gunpowders before 1000 A.D.[7] This was many years before the gunpowder became known in the Western world. The ancient Sanskrit writings from India translated by the East India Company in 1776 suggest that the knowledge of gunpowder existed in India almost 500 years before that date.[13] Many modern researchers, however, are not convinced that gunpowder was known as a propellant before the 13th century. Despite all claims, it can be said that it is not proved beyond doubt which individual invented gunpowder and realized its capabilities. Even the time and the place of invention are not certain.

Blackpowder

The oldest explosive known to man is blackpowder. It was known and used in Europe by the 13th century.[3] At that time it was composed of a mixture of charcoal (15%), sulphur (10%) and saltpeter (75%). (The powder first used in the United States consisted 15.6 per cent of charcoal, 10.4 per cent of sulphur and 74 per cent of saltpeter.) The mixture, ground to fine dust, called "serpentine," was used until the middle of the 16th century. After this, "corned" powder that was more stable replaced "serpentine." This powder, however, exploded all at

1

once and frequently led to accidents. Many modifications of blackpowder were developed, some containing potassium nitrate and others sodium nitrate. All these blackpowders had the great disadvantage of producing smoke and causing fouling. When they burned, rapid oxidation of charcoal and sulphur produced carbon monoxide, carbon dioxide and nitrogen gases and solid products such as potassium carbonate, potassium sulphate and potassium sulphides. These solid products with carbon formed over 50 per cent of the weight of the powder.

Smokeless Powder

The shortcomings of blackpowder, namely smoking and fouling, led to the replacement of this powder by smokeless powder. The basic ingredient in the development of smokeless powder was nitrocellulose. When nitrocellulose was reduced with suitable solvents to a homogeneous solid, it burned only at the surface and did not explode at once. This made it a usable propellant. The first step in the production of nitrocellulose was the addition of nitric acid to cellulose fibers. Cellulose nitrate thus produced is an explosive substance creating carbon monoxide, carbon dioxide, nitrogen, hydrogen and steam. This process of nitration eventually led to the making of acceptable smokeless powder. The first successful use of smokeless powders in rifles was developed by M. Vieille in 1884 for the French Government.[14] Three years later, Alfred Nobel invented a smokeless powder called Ballistite with the composition of nitroglycerine (40%) and nitrocellulose (60%).

Historically, smokeless powder was developed first for shotguns. According to Harrison, Captain E. Schultze of the Prussian Army made the first successful use of smokeless powder in shotguns in 1864.[13] The powder was made of nitroglignin. Better smokeless powders were, of course, produced later for shotguns by the Hercules and duPont companies.

In the early 1890's, smokeless powder had replaced blackpowder as propellant and by the year 1900 it was being used in most military rifles. In the United States, the E. I. duPont de Nemours and Company were the principal manufacturers of smokeless powders. Their powders had only nitrocellulose as the base constituent. In the early 20th century, the Hercules Powder Company produced a double-base smokeless powder with nitroglycerine and nitrocellulose.

Smokeless powder gained in use because its components contain adequate oxygen to allow it to burn in a gun chamber without the need for additional oxygen from outside sources. When the powder is ignited in the gun, the heat and gas in the chamber increase the pressure, leading to more heat, burning and explosion.

GUNS

Earliest Weapons

As soon as gunpowder was invented, guns arrived on the scene. The first guns developed were designed to be fired from mounts or carriages. By modern terminology they could be considered artillery. The development of the handgun almost paralleled the development of the cannon. During the first half of the 14th century, several different small arms were developed. These were at the time called hand cannons. They consisted simply of iron or brass tubes open at one end and with a hole on top of the closed end. The cylinders or tubes were about 9 inches long. The earliest evidence of the actual use of small arms comes from Italy. The first practical pistols, single-shot wheellocks, originated in Germany about 1520.[5]

Rifling originated in the matchlock era as a means of facilitating loading and cleaning. It is not known whether the invention of rifling occurred in Germany or Austria, but the earliest-dated rifled firearms in use between 1493 and 1508 bore the arms of the German Emperor Maximilian I. There is evidence of the use of curved rifling in the late 15th and early 16th century. The military first used the rifled weapons in Denmark during the period 1577–1648.[13]

According to records of the British Royal Society dated March 2, 1663, the principle of the semi-automatic weapon was an English discovery.[13] However, the real practical improvement of the semi-automatic rifle was made by an American, Hiram Maxim in the years 1881–1883. Maxim is, therefore, considered the father of modern automatic weapons. Josserand and Stevenson believe that the first automatic pistol actually produced, in 1887, was French.[5]

The first of the pistols were delicate muzzle-loaders with one or two barrels. These pistols fired a musket ball in front of the powder charge.

Loading of the gun at the muzzle was soon found to be impractical for soldiers in combat. Therefore, attempts to produce guns that could be loaded at the breech and that could fire several times were made. One of these first efforts in the 16th century produced breech-loaders with separate chambers that could first be loaded and then inserted into the breech. Further progress in the direction of breech-loading led to the making of a pistol that consisted of several barrels arranged around an axis. In the early and mid 18th century, these guns used by travellers for defense were formidable handguns with a 6- to 8-inch barrel capable of firing a ball weighing half an ounce or more. The earliest of these handguns was an over-under type with the barrel assembly rotated manually after the first shot to bring the loaded lower barrel up for firing. A pair of over-under barrels allowed four shots to be fired individually and successively without stopping to reload. A few guns with as many as 15 barrels or more appeared in the Middle Ages. However, the majority of these pistols had less than six barrels and most of them had about half the caliber of modern single- or double-barreled pistols. These ancient guns with multiple barrels are today known as *Pepperbox* pistols. With various improvements pistols reached their functional peak in the latter half of the 18th century. Although in the earlier models the barrel assembly had to be rotated by hand for each shot, the work of Joseph Land of London in 1830 led to mechanization of the barrel assembly's rotation.

The disadvantage of the popular pepperbox pistols was that the automatic revolving of the barrel with the pulling of the trigger and the rising of the cock made aims difficult. Samuel Colt solved the problem of accurate aiming in 1835 by developing a revolver in which a cylinder containing the chambers revolved but the barrel of the gun remained stationary. He achieved this by introducing internal mechanisms that revolved the cylinder and locked it in line with the barrel after each shot was fired. Although a significant improvement, the Colt pistol was not entirely free from fault. Its great disadvantage was the reloading; the charging of each chamber with powder and bullet from the front of the cylinder and the placing of a small percussion cap on the nipple of each chamber at the rear was a slow process.

As far as the earliest American arms are concerned, not much is known. The Pilgrims and the Puritans used cheap matchlocks. However, the flintlocks had already gone through advanced development in Europe, and the German settlers brought these to America. The original rifles brought to this country were heavy, large-bore firearms with short barrels. Later, lighter and quicker-loading rifles were developed. Various committees set up in 1775 in the first 13 colonies authorized the use of smoothbore muskets with calibers varying from 0.72 to 0.80 as the official arms of the militia units of the United States. The first official musket was the Charleville Flintlock, used by the French army. The first Mauser rifle for practical use was patented in the United States in 1868. This weapon was widely used after its development.

The first French revolver of pepperbox type was the Lefaucheux, produced in 1851. Immediately after its production, there came into existence many revolvers with pinfire cartridges. The revolver achieved its apex of development by 1900; after this, the improvements made were not significant. The early 1900's saw the introduction of 0.25 caliber automatics such as the Browning and the Manufrance. Some of the finest one-handed weapons, Colt 0.45 Government Model and the Luger, appeared before the first World War.

Ignition Systems in Ancient Guns. The ignition system in ancient firearm was called "lock." The earliest firearms, cannon locks, were fired with the help of a hot iron or a lighted coal held near the powder placed over a touchhole. In the 14th century, the powder was ignited by introducing a burning stick or wire through the hole. Around 1400, the touchhole, which used to be at the top of the barrel, was shifted to the side of the barrel to facilitate ignition of the powder in an attached pan.

The first of the ignition systems was the *matchlock*. It made use of a hemp fiber treated with saltpeter and other substances to make it slow-burning. This fiber was twisted and tied by a thread to retain the twists. It was placed in a split of a metal piece pivoted at the side of the stock ready for ignition. Once ignited at its free end, it burned at the rate of 3 to 5 inches per hour. There is no certainty about the date or place of origin of the first matchlock but it appears that it was probably invented during the latter half of the 15th century.

The need to avoid the use of live coals, burning matches or hemp fibers led to the invention of the *wheellock*. This primitive form of ignition system uses the simple principle of our modern-day cigarette lighters. A steel wheel was used to produce sparks. The spinning of the serrated wheel against a flint with push and pull motions created showers of sparks. These sparks ignited the priming powder, and through the touchhole the flash fire reached the powder charge in the priming chamber. As is the case with the matchlock, there is also uncertainty about the date of development of the wheellock; some people, however, believe that the wheellock was invented in Germany in the early years of the 16th century.[8]

The *flintlock* ignition system superseded the wheellock. A simple mechanical fire striking lock called *snaphaunce* replaced the wheel mechanism. This snaphaunce, and an iron right-angle pan cover hinged over the priming pan, constituted the flintlock. The hinged piece was struck by the cock, which threw the hinged cover back. This exposed the priming powder in the pan, and as that happened the sparks produced by the scraping of flint along the iron went down into the priming powder.

Another ignition system, called the *percussion system*, was invented by Alexander John Forsyth in 1807. He patented a compound that would explode if struck. The use of mercury fulminate to produce a flash for setting off ignition led to the eventual making of the famous percussion cap by Joshua Shaw in 1814. The percussion cap was made of copper or iron with a cavity to contain the percussion compound. To fire the weapon, one had to place the cap on a conical projection from the barrel. When the hammer struck the cap, a flash would be produced, and this flash would enter the bore and set off the charge. It took several years before the flintlock system was replaced in Europe by the more convenient percussion cap. By the middle of the 19th century, it was commonly used in military arms. The United States continued to use the percussion cap system in its military arms through the Civil War of 1861–65.

CARTRIDGES

In the earlier guns one of the drawbacks was the time spent in loading the gun. An improvement in the safety and speed of loading was the invention of cartridges. The word "cartridge" is derived from the Latin word "charta," which means paper. The first of the cartridges were in the form of a powder charge wrapped in paper and appeared in the latter half of the 16th century. The bullet had to be loaded separately. By 1700, the powder and the bullet were wrapped together in paper for easy loading. Later, many different materials such as cloth, rubber and metal were used to wrap the bullet and the powder until the self-contained cartridge encased in metal or metal and paper was evolved. The first self-contained cartridge was produced in 1835 by Lefaucheux in France. In the United States, the first metal-cased cartridge was developed by Horace Smith and Daniel Wesson in 1857. These two men are given credit for further improvement in later cartridges containing their own primer.

Pinfire Cartridge

The first of the cartridges was of the pinfire type. The percussion cap was mounted in the side of the base with a pin above the base protruding through the case. A hammer blow would drive the pin into the cap, explode it and set off the charge. These pinfire cartridges led to the development of a series of better cartridges. The original forms have been out of production for years.

Rimfire Cartridge

The next cartridge type to be developed was the rimfire type, and in the 1860's pinfire cartridges were supplanted by rimfire cartridges. In the rimfire type, the firing pin hit the top of the case and crushed the metal to detonate the priming. Smith and Wesson introduced rimfire cartridges with a black powder and priming compound. The rimfire cartridge also has fallen into disuse today.

Centerfire Cartridge

This cartridge came into use in 1870. In most of the center-fire cartridges there was a rimmed or rimless case. The powder was placed in the center of the base and was crushed against a rigid perforated anvil by the action of the hammer.

Various modifications followed. The cartridges developed were either straight, tapered or bottleneck, and their head forms were either rimmed, semi-rimless, rimless, rebated-rimless or belted rimless. The rimless cartridge was first manufactured in the United States in 1892.

SUMMARY

This chapter is a short review of some of the salient historical firearm developments. Modern crime investigators will rarely, if ever, be involved in the problems of identification of ancient weapons. Therefore, inclusion of details about those firearms is not justified in a volume of this nature. For information on the 19th-century firearms, the investigator is referred to many of the outstanding works such as those by Blair (1968)[1], Gould (1894)[2], Hatcher (1927)[4], Mathews (1962)[6], Sell (1963)[10], Smith (1948)[11], Smith and Bellah (1965)[12], Taylerson (1965)[15], and Taylerson (1971).[16] One bibliography, listing almost 3,000 gun books, is of great value to researchers.[9]

REFERENCES

1. Blair, C.: Pistols of the World. London, B. T. Batsford, 1968.
2. Gould, A. C.: Modern American Pistols and Revolvers. Boston, Bradlee Whidden, 1894.
3. Harrison, E. H.: Blackpowder. *In* The N.R.A. Handloader's Guide. Washington, D.C., National Rifle Association, 1969.
4. Hatcher, J. S.: Pistols and Revolvers and Their Use. Delaware, Small-Arms Technical Publishing, 1927.
5. Josserand, M. H., and Stevenson, J. A.: Pistols, Revolvers and Ammunition. New York, Crown Publishers, 1972.
6. Mathews, J. H.: Firearms Identification. Madison, University of Wisconsin Press, 1962.
7. Partington, J. K.: A History of Greek Fire and Gunpowder. Cited by Smith, W. H. B., and Smith, J. E.: Small Arms of the World, ed. 10. Harrisburg, Stackpole, 1973.
8. Peterson, H. L., and Logan, H. C.: The Development of Firearms. *In* The N.R.A. Handloader's Guide. Washington, D.C., National Rifle Association, 1969.

9. Riling, R.: Guns and Shooting. A Bibliography. New York, Greenburg, 1951.
10. Sell, De W. E.: Collector's Guide to American Cartridge Handguns. Harrisburg, Stackpole, 1963.
11. Smith, W. H. B.: Small Arms of the World. Harrisburg, Military Service Publishing, 1948.
12. Smith, W. H. B., and Bellah, K.: Book of Pistols and Revolvers. Harrisburg, Stackpole, 1965.
13. Smith, W. H. B., and Smith, J. E.: The Book of Rifles, ed. 4. Harrisburg, Stackpole, 1972.
14. ———: Small Arms of the World. ed. 10. Harrisburg, Stackpole, 1973.
15. Taylerson, A. W. F.: The Revolver, 1865–1888. London, Herbert Jenkins, 1965.
16. ———: The Revolver, 1889–1914. New York, Crown Publishers, 1971.

2

Modern Firearms and Ammunition: Basic Information

Numerous makes and models of guns with varied characteristics exist. In general, these guns can be divided into two groups: rifled weapons and smoothbored guns.

RIFLED WEAPONS

Rifled guns are of two types: long-barreled shoulder arms (rifles) and short-barreled handguns (pistols and revolvers). These guns bear a number of parallel but spiral lands (projecting ridges) and grooves (depressed spirals between the lands) on the interior of the barrel from the breech to the muzzle, referred to as rifling. The rifling causes a spiraling motion of the bullet and imparts gyroscopic steadiness to it during its flight. The diameter of a gun bore is the distance between the two opposite lands. This distance, expressed in hundreths of an inch, is called *caliber* (Fig. 2-1). The term caliber is also applied to designate the diameter of a bullet.

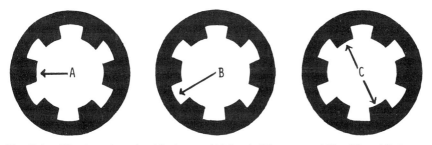

Fig. 2-1. The interior of a rifled gun: (A) land, (B) groove, (C) caliber (distance between two opposite lands).

9

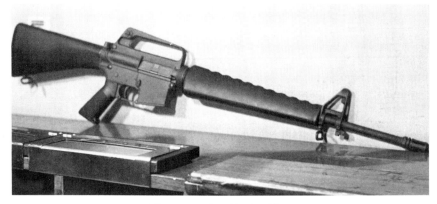

Fig. 2-2. An AR-15 rifle.

Rifles

Many varieties of rifles are available. They may be single shot or multiple shot weapons. Single shot rifles are not common. Double rifles, which are made in Europe, are also not common in the United States. A gun with a combination of a shotgun and a rifle called combination rifle is also made, but such a rifle is rare in the United States. By law, all rifles have to have barrels at least 16 inches long. Common rifles can be classified on the basis of their action type.

Bolt-Action Rifles. This is a commonly used type, popular with shooters because of its accuracy. These rifles offer many varieties of calibers and loads. Commonly used American bolt-action center-fire rifles are Smith and Wesson Model MB, Winchester Models 70, 760 and M1898, Harrington and Richardson Model 330, Remington Model 700BDL and Mossberg Model 800D.

Lever-Action Rifles. Many lever-action rifles with twenty-four-inch barrels are available. These include 0.243, 0.284, 0.308 and 0.30/30 Winchester, 0.250/3000 and 0.300 Savage, 0.35 Remington and 0.44 Magnum.

Slide-Action Rifles. Remington and Savage make slide-action rifles, which make rapid fire possible with quick sighting.

Automatic Rifles. These are the fastest of the guns automatically loading and cocking with each pull of the trigger.

For target practice, the most popular of the rifles are Winchester Model 70 and Remington 540XB.

Some of the basic types of rifles most frequently used by criminals are 0.22 caliber Winchester Model 290 semi-automatic, 0.30-30 caliber Marlin Model 336 lever-action, 0.30-30 caliber Winchester Model 94 lever-action, 0.22 caliber Winchester Model 69 bolt-action, 0.30 caliber U.S.

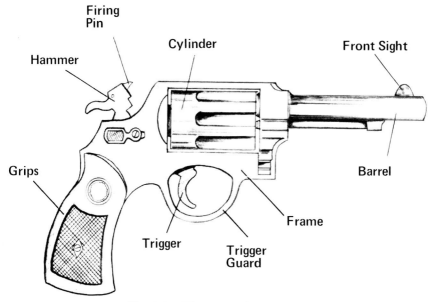

Fig. 2-3.   The parts of a revolver.

M-1 carbine, 0.223 caliber Colt AR-15 (M-16), 0.30 caliber British SMLE, 0.30 caliber U.S. M-1 (Garand).[2]

M-16 Rifle.   The M-16 rifle (AR-15), although a combat weapon, is finding its ways into civilian life and is sometimes used in crime. It is a lightweight (6.5 pounds without magazine) semi-automatic or fully automatic shoulder weapon (Fig. 2-2). It is a high velocity (muzzle velocity 3250 feet per second) weapon capable of causing massive tissue damage out of proportion to the size of the bullet.

Handguns

Handguns are divided into two classes: the revolvers and the pistols. Both can be further classified as "Colt type," which have six lands and grooves and a left hand rifling twist, and the "Smith and Wesson type" which have five lands and grooves and a right-hand rifling twist. Guns with greater or smaller number of lands and grooves with different directions of twist are also made.

Revolvers.   Of the short-barreled rifled weapons, the revolver is recognized by the way the ammunition is carried to the breech. A metal drum, having spaces for cartridges, revolves each time the trigger is released, bringing into position the next live cartridge for firing. Various parts of a revolver are illustrated in Figure 2-3.

There are two main types of revolvers: single action and double ac-

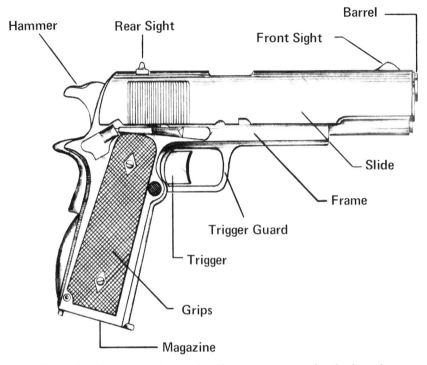

Hammer   Rear Sight   Front Sight   Barrel

Slide

Frame

Trigger Guard

Trigger

Grips

Magazine

Fig. 2-4.   An automatic pistol with a magazine under the breech.

tion. In the single action revolver, the hammer has to be pulled back and cocked before the gun can be fired. In the double action type, the revolver cocks itself when the trigger is pulled. Most modern revolvers are the double action type.

The center-fire revolvers carry up to six shots in their metal drums, but some of the 0.22 caliber rim-fires take up to nine shots in the revolving cylinders. Revolvers can also handle magnum loads.

Examples of commonly used revolvers are 0.22 caliber Iver Johnson, 0.28 caliber Smith and Wesson and 0.45 caliber Webley-Fosberry. One of the most commonly used revolvers is the 0.38 Special used by police.

Pistols.   The automatics or automatic pistols have cartridges placed in a metal clip-type box (magazine) under the breech instead of in a revolving cylinder (Fig. 2-4). Each time the trigger is pulled the bullet in the breech is fired and the spent cartridge is automatically ejected. At the same time a spring mechanism pushes the next live cartridge into the breech ready to be fired. Although these handguns are called automatics, they are not truly automatic. In a really automatic gun, once the trigger is pulled, repeated shots will be fired with automatic cocking. In pistols that are really semi-automatic, the trigger has to be pulled

Fig. 2-5. The components of a cartridge.

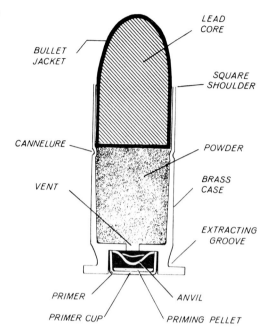

LEAD CORE

BULLET JACKET

SQUARE SHOULDER

CANNELURE

POWDER

VENT

BRASS CASE

EXTRACTING GROOVE

PRIMER

ANVIL

PRIMER CUP

PRIMING PELLET

each time a shot needs to be fired. The pull of the trigger automatically ejects the empty cartridge case, reloads another shot and cocks the gun.

Automatic pistols are common in 0.22 caliber. They are also made in other calibers, except for Magnum loads. The automatics with center-fire loadings are made to take up to nine shots. The 0.22 caliber pistols can take up to ten shots in their magazine. The 9 mm automatic made by Browning has a 13-shot capacity.

Among the pistols, the 0.22 caliber Webley and Scott, 0.25 caliber Colt and the 0.45 caliber Colt are commonly used. Some of the handguns that are commonly used to commit crimes are 0.22 caliber RG-10 2½-inch barrel revolver, 0.22 caliber Ruger 5½-inch barrel "single six" revolver, 0.22 caliber high standard semi-automatic pistol, 0.25 caliber Colt "pocket automatic" pistols, 0.32 caliber Harrington and Richardson 3¼-inch barrel revolver, 0.32 caliber Beretta Model 1934 semi-automatic pistol, 0.357 Magnum Smith and Wesson "combat magnum" revolver, 0.38 caliber Smith and Wesson revolver (Spanish-made copy), 0.38 caliber Smith and Wesson 2-inch barrel "chief's special" revolver, 0.38 caliber Colt Model 1908 semi-automatic pistol, 9MM Smith and Wesson Model 39 pistol, 9MM German P-38 Walther pistol, 0.45 caliber U.S. Model 1911-A1 pistol.[2]

Saturday Night Special.   The phrase "Saturday Night Special" originated in Detroit in the early 1960's. When Detroiters bought guns

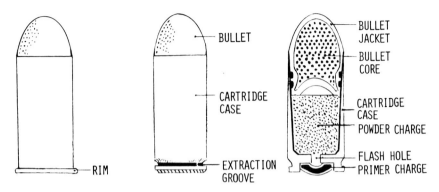

Fig. 2-6. Cartridges with rim and groove.

from Toledo, Ohio to satisfy their Saturday night passions, the Detroit law enforcement agents started to refer to these guns as "Saturday Night Specials."[5] These were cheap, substandard imported guns that could easily be bought in Ohio at the time. Most of these Specials are low caliber (0.22, 0.25 or 0.32 caliber) guns.

The 1968 Gun Control Act contributed substantially to the increase of Saturday Night Specials in the United States. The Act prohibited the entry of all foreign military surplus weapons and import of any guns that failed to meet certain criteria. However, it did not prohibit the import of gun parts. As a result, large amounts of gun parts arrived in the country, and the assembly of miscellaneous parts formed a flood of Saturday Night Specials. Sawing off of barrels of imported guns resulted in another variety of Specials.

There are so many varieties of Specials that it is not possible to say what truly is a Saturday Night Special. It is estimated that about two million Specials are put on the market each year in the United States.

AMMUNITION FOR RIFLED WEAPONS

The ammunition for a rifled firearm is a cartridge. It consists of a cartridge case, usually made of brass, primer, powder charge and bullet (Fig. 2-5.) The cartridge cases are designed with four types of bases: rimmed (Fig. 2-6), semi-rimmed, rimless and belted.

The primer is a percussion component placed in a receptacle at the base of the cartridge. Its function is to convert mechanical energy to chemical energy. When the trigger is pulled, the firing pin is driven into the primer, which ignites. The flash fire passes through a flash hole in the cartridge base to reach the powder charge. Depending on where the primer is placed in relation to the base of the cartridge and how it is

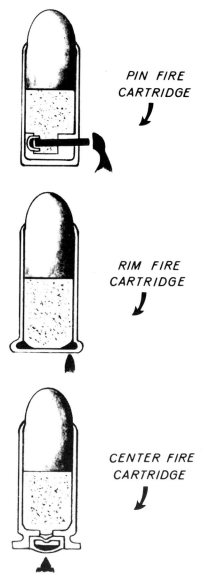

PIN FIRE
CARTRIDGE

RIM FIRE
CARTRIDGE

CENTER FIRE
CARTRIDGE

Fig. 2-7.   Three types of cartridges.

ignited, the cartridges are termed pinfire, rimfire or centerfire type (Fig. 2-7). In the rimfire cartridge the primer is placed in a small rim at the base of the case. In the centerfire ammunition the primer is in the base of the cartridge.

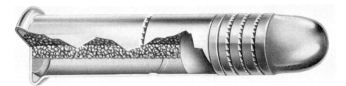

Fig. 2-8. Long Rifle cartridge (Courtesy of Winchester-Western).

The powder charge consists of nitrocellulose or nitrocellulose combined with nitroglycerin. Rapid burning of the powder causes high pressure, which drives the bullet out of the mouth of the case and out of the barrel of the gun.

The bullets are variously shaped: flat nose, round nose, hollow point, spine and spitzer. Modern pistol and revolver bullets are of two kinds: solid metal bullets made of lead alloyed with tin or antimony, and composite bullets made of a central core of lead with a jacket of harder metal. In the jacketed bullets the lead core is either partially or completely covered with an alloy usually containing copper. Semijacketed bullets are partially covered; the alloy jacket is thick at the base but thins gradually toward the point of the bullet. Modern jacketed bullets used in rifles have jackets made of steel, cupro-nickel, copper-zinc-nickel alloy, copper-zinc alloy or copper-zinc-tin alloy.

Common 0.22 caliber cartridges in rimfire type are Short, Long, and Long Rifle, the latter being the most popular (Fig. 2-8). Details of various cartridges manufactured in the U.S. are summarized in Table 2-1.

SMOOTHBORE WEAPONS: SHOTGUNS

Shotguns are smoothbore weapons; that is, the inside wall of the barrel is not rifled. There are different types of shotguns:

1. Single barrel shotgun: the single barrel break-open shotgun is a basic model.

2. Double barrel break-open shotgun: there are various types of double barrel shotguns. Some have barrels set side-by-side and the others have over-and-under barrels. The side-by-side double barrel shotguns have always been popular. Some double-barrel shotguns are made in the U.S., but most of them are foreign made. Double-barrel shotguns

(Text continued on p. 20)

Table 2-1. Standard Commercial U.S. Cartridges for Rifle, Pistol, and Revolver

Cartridge Nomenclature	Chambered In†			Approximate Groove Diameter of Fired Bullet (in.)	Muzzle Velocity (ft. per sec.)
	Pistol	Revolver	Rifle		
.22 Short* HV	+	+	+	.217 to .223	1125
.22 Long* HV	+	+	+	.217 to .223	1240
.22 Long Rifle* HV	+	+	+	.217 to .223	1335
.22 Winchester Auto*			+	.217 to .223	1055
.22 W.R.F.* HV			+	.226	1450
.22 WMR* (Magnum)	+	+		.223	1550
.22 WMR* (Magnum)			+	.223	2000
.22 Remington Jet Magnum		+	+	.222	2460
.218 Bee			+	.224	2860
.219 Zipper			+	.224	3110
.221 Remington Fireball	+			.224	2650
.22 Hornet			+	.224	2690
.220 Swift			+	.224	4110
.22 Savage HP			+	.227	2800
.22-250 Remington			+	.224	3760
.222 Remington			+	.224	3200
.222 Remington Magnum			+	.224	3300
.223 Remington HV (5.56 mm)			+	.224	3300
.225 Winchester			+	.224	3650
.243 Winchester HV			+	.243	3500
					3070
6 mm Remington			+	.243	3190
.244 Remington HV			+	.243	3500
					3200
.25 ACP	+			.250	810
.25-20			+	.257	1460
					2250
.250 Savage			+	.257	3030
					2820
.25-35			+	.257	2300
.25 Remington			+	.257	2320
.256 Winchester Magnum	+		+	.257	2800
					2350
.257 Roberts			+		3200
				.257	2650
.264 Winchester Magnum			+	.264	3700
					3200
.270 Winchester			+	.277	3580
					2800
.280 Remington			+	.284	3140
					2770

*Indicates rimfire; others, centerfire.
†Indicates "yes, Chambered".
(Modified from Camps, F. E. (ed.): Gradwohl's Legal Medicine. Bristol, John Wright & Sons, 1968.)

(Table continued, overleaf)

Table 2-1.   Standard Commercial U.S. Cartridges for
Rifle, Pistol, and Revolver (Continued)

	Chambered In†			Approximate Groove Diameter of Fired Bullet (in.)	Muzzle Velocity (ft. per sec.)
Cartridge Nomenclature	Pistol	Revolver	Rifle		
.284 Winchester			+	.284	3200
					2900
7 mm Remington Magnum			+	.284	3260
					3020
7 mm Mauser (7 x 57)			+	.284	2490
.30 Mauser (7.63)	+			.302	1410
.30 Luger (7.65 mm)	+			.301	1220
.30 Carbine, U.S.			+	.308	1980
.30-30 Winchester			+	.308	2410
					2220
.30 Remington			+	.308	2220
.308 Winchester (7.62 mm.)			+	.308	3340
					2450
.30-40 Krag			+	.308	2470
					2200
.30-06			+	.308	3420
					2410
.300 Savage			+	.308	2670
					1980
.300 Holland & Holland			+	.308	3190
Magnum					2620
.300 Winchester Magnum			+	.308	3400
					3070
.303 British			+	.311	2540
					2180
.303 Savage			+	.308	2140
					1980
.32 New Police		+		.312	680
.32 ACP (7.65 mm)	+			.312	960
.32 S & W		+		.312	680
.32 S & W Long	+			.312	705
					2100
.32-20 Winchester		+	+	.310	1290
					1030
.32-40 Winchester			+	.320	1440
.32 Winchester Special			+	.320	2280
.32 Remington			+	.320	2220
8 mm Lebel			+	.322	2640
8 mm Mauser (8 x 57 mm)			+	.322	2570
.338 Winchester Magnum			+	.338	3000
					2700
.348 Winchester			+	.348	2530
					2350
.35 Remington			+	.358	2400
					2210

Table 2-1. Standard Commercial U.S. Cartridges for Rifle, Pistol, and Revolver (Continued)

Cartridge Nomenclature	Chambered In† Pistol	Chambered In† Revolver	Chambered In† Rifle	Approximate Groove Diameter of Fired Bullet (in.)	Muzzle Velocity (ft. per sec.)
.35 Winchester			+	.357	2160
.350 Remington Magnum			+	.358	2410
.351 Winchester selfloading			+	.351	1850
.357 Magnum			+	.357	1550
.358 Winchester			+	.358	2530
					2250
9 mm Luger	+			.356	1120
.375 Holland & Holland			+	.375	2740
Magnum					2550
.38 S & W		+		.354	685
.38 Special		+		.357	1320
					730
.38 New Police		+		.357	680
.38 Short Colt		+		.375	730
.38 Long Colt		+		.357	730
.38-40 Winchester		+	+	.400	1330
					775
.38 Super	+			.354	1280
.38 ACP	+			.354	1040
.380 ACP	+			.354	955
.38-55			+	.376	1320
.401 Winchester selfloading			+	.407	2190
.405 Winchester			+	.413	2260
.41 Long Colt		+		.402	730
.41 Remington Magnum		+		.411	1150
.44 Special		+		.427	755
.44 Remington Magnum		+	+	.430	1850
					1470
.44-40		+	+	.425	1310
					975
.444 Marlin			+	.430	2400
.45 ACP	+	+		.451	1140
					850
.45 Auto Rim		+		.443	810
.45-70 Government			+	.457	1320
.458 Winchester Magnum			+	.458	2125
.45-90			+	.457	1530

*Indicates rimfire; others, centerfire.
†Indicates "yes, Chambered".
(Modified from Camps, F. E. (ed.): Gradwohl's Legal Medicine. Bristol, John Wright & Sons, 1968.)

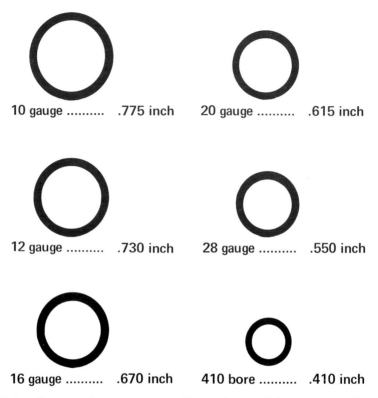

10 gauge .... .775 inch   20 gauge .... .615 inch

12 gauge .... .730 inch   28 gauge .... .550 inch

16 gauge .... .670 inch   410 bore .... .410 inch

Fig. 2-9. Common shotgun gauges with *actual* sizes of the diameters of barrels and their decimal equivalents (Courtesy of Winchester-Western).

may have different chokes in the two barrels and they may be fired with one or two triggers. Some are equipped with extractors or ejectors. In the over-and-under type, one barrel is above the other with a single sight. The lower barrel usually has a lesser choke.

3. Bolt action shotgun: these shotguns carry extra shells in the magazine, which is fitted into the breech. The action of the bolt ejects the fired shell and loads the next one.

4. Lever action shotgun: this is a gun with a lever that serves as a trigger guard, and, when it is swung down, it ejects the fired shell and loads the next shot.

5. Pump action shotgun: this is one of the most popular shotguns in the U.S. It can fire as fast as the autoloaders. In this gun there is a cylinder type magazine which can contain shells lying end-to-end in a horizontal row beneath the barrel. Pump guns can be loaded with up to six shells.

Table 2-2. Types and Degrees of Choke

Choke	Degree of Choke: Percentage of Pellets Within a 30-inch Circle when Fired from 40 Yards
Skeet	30–35 per cent
Cylinder bore	35–45 per cent
Improved Cylinder	45–55 per cent
Modified	55–65 per cent
Full choke	65–75 per cent

6. Autoloading shotgun: in this popular shotgun, a pull on the trigger not only fires the shot and ejects the shell but also reloads the next shot and locks it for refiring. Although they are referred to as automatic shotguns, they are actually semi-automatic.

The shotguns commonly used by criminals include the 12-gauge single barrel sawed-off shotgun, 12-gauge Browning "automatic 5" shotgun, 12-gauge Mossberg bolt action shotgun, Mossberg pump action shotgun with variable choke, 20-gauge Winchester model 12 sawed-off shotgun and Savage pump action shotgun with variable choke.[2]

Gauge of a Shotgun

Shotguns are usually designated by the diameter of the barrel (bore); the unit of measure is the *gauge* and it is determined by the number of solid balls of pure lead, each with the diameter of the barrel, that can be prepared from one pound of lead. If 12 balls can be made from one pound of lead, each ball exactly fitting the inside of the barrel of a shotgun, the gun is called a 12-gauge or 12-bore shotgun. Each lead ball for a 12-gauge shot should weigh $1/12$ of a pound. This system of nomenclature does not apply to the 0.410-gauge shotgun in which the bore or the gauge is measured in the thousandths of an inch. The gauge of a shotgun is thus a measure similar to the caliber of a rifled weapon.

The 12-gauge shotgun is the most commonly used shotgun. The 16-gauge gun is lighter than the 12-gauge one and is easier to handle. The 0.410-gauge shotgun is the lightest. Common bore gauges with the actual sizes of the diameters of shotgun barrels and their decimal equivalent are listed in Figure 2-9. The 10-gauge shotgun is the biggest bore allowed by federal law for hunting, but some 8-gauge shotguns with bore diameter of 0.835 inch are also made. It should be pointed out that the measurements of the same gauges in guns made by different manufacturers are not always identical. For instance, a 12-gauge shotgun

CLOSING
WAD

SHOT

FILLER
WADS

OVER-
POWDER
WAD

PROPELLANT
POWDER

BATTERY
CUP

PRIMER
CUP

Fig. 2-10.   The structure of a shotgun shell.

PAPER
TUBE

METAL
BASE

ANVIL

PRIMING

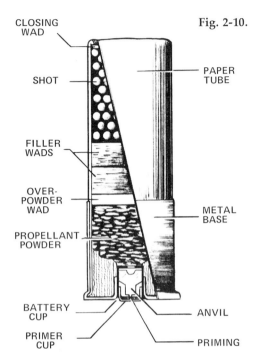

made by one manufacturer may vary by as much as 0.025 inch from a 12-gauge shotgun produced by another company.[4]

Modern shotgun barrels measure 26, 28 and 30 inches in length. A shotgun may be equipped with a simple sighting aid of a colored bead mounted on the barrel or a more useful scope sight or biocular sight.

Choke of a Shotgun

The choke is the boring of the barrel so that the muzzle end of the barrel has a diameter smaller than the rest of the barrel. In other words, the degree of constriction at the muzzle of a shotgun barrel is called the choke. The choke is designed to keep the shot together over a longer distance. Choke is determined by the percentage of pellets that strike within a 30-inch circle when fired from a shotgun from a distance of 40 yards. There are various degrees of choke; these are classified in Table 2-2.

Chokes can be varied in different ways. Popular devices to vary chokes are Win-Choke (Winchester Arms Co.) and Poly-Choke (Poly-Choke Co.). In the former, there are three interchangeable tubes of different constrictions that can be inserted with a wrench; in the latter, choke can be varied simply by turning a sleeve with the fingers. Only a

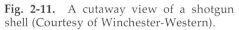

Fig. 2-11. A cutaway view of a shotgun shell (Courtesy of Winchester-Western).

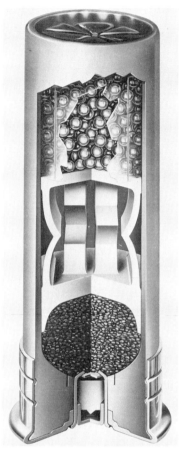

small change is needed to alter the choke. For instance, in a standard 0.729-inch bore of a 12-gauge shotgun a constriction of 0.035 inch will make it a full choke barrel.[3]

S<small>HOTGUN</small> A<small>MMUNITION</small>

Shotgun ammunition consists of shells or cartridges with pellets or slugs. Early shotgun shells were composed of brass shell, brass cup, primer, base wad, powder, shot, over powder wad, filler wads and overshot wad. The primer consisted of a cup (to hold chemicals), an anvil and a flash hole. The shot was made of lead, and arsenic was added for roundness and antimony for hardening. The shell cases used to be made of brass only.

In recent times, many changes have occurred in the composition of

Table 2-3.   Size and Weight of Pellets Used in Shotguns

Shot Number	Diameter of Pellet (in inches)	Number of Pellets Per Ounce	Weight of Each Pellet (in grams)
12	0.05	2385	0.0118
10	0.07	870	0.0325
9	0.08	585	0.0471
8	0.09	410	0.0691
7½	0.095	350	0.0810
6	0.11	225	0.1260
5	0.12	170	0.1667
4	0.13	135	0.2100
2	0.15	90	0.3150
BB	0.18	50	0.5670

shotgun shells. Polyethylene plastic shells, for instance, came into use in 1960. Laminated paper attached to a brass base is also used to make shell cases. The components within the shells have also changed. In modern shotgun shells, plastic shot sleeve, plastic wads and crimp are used.

In a typical modern shotgun shell, the primer reaches up to the base. Around the primer is a wad, about 9/16 inch thick, made of compressed paper. This acts as a gas seal. Ahead of this wad is powder charge, in front of which is another wad called powder wad. Filler pads occupy some space ahead of the powder wad. The shot placed in front of the filler wad is held in place by crimping the edge of the shell mouth (Figs. 2-10, 2-11).

How is the shot fired with such a shell? When the trigger is pulled, the firing pin activates the primer. The flash thus produced passes through the flash-hole and ignites the powder. Increased pressures of gas hurl the wads forward. The wads blast the shot out of the shell by

Table 2-4.   Size, Number and Weight of Pellets Used in
Various Buckshots

Buckshot Number	Diameter of Pellet (in inches)	Number of Pellets Per Shell	Number of Pellets Per Pound
4	0.24	27	340
3	0.25	20	300
1	0.30	16	175
0	0.32	12	145
00	0.33	9	130

Standard Shot Chart

No.	12	11	10	9	8	7½	6	5	4	2
DIAMETER IN INCHES	.05	.06	.07	.08	.09	.095	.11	.12	.13	.15
APPROXIMATE NUMBER OF PELLETS TO THE OUNCE	2385	1380	870	585	410	350	225	170	135	90

	Air Rifle	BB	No.4 Buck	No.3 Buck	No.1 Buck	No.0 Buck	No.00
DIAMETER IN INCHES	.175	.18	.24	.25	.30	.32	.33
NUMBER TO THE OUNCE / APPROXIMATE NUMBER TO THE POUND	55	50	340	300	175	145	130

Fig. 2-12. A chart showing shot diameter in inches for various shot sizes and approximate number of pellets per ounce with diameters of buckshot and number of shots per pound (Courtesy of Winchester-Western).

uncrimping it. Carried to variable distances with the shot are flame, smoke and unburned gunpowder.

Shotgun barrels are constructed to conform to the length of the shell. The shells used in the shotguns are either 2¾ or 3 inches long. These measurements do not refer to the length of intact shells; they represent the length of opened shells with unrolled crimp. Thus, an unopened or unfired shell may be about ½ inch shorter than its designated length. The ammunition for 0.410 gauge shotgun includes 2½-inch shell with half an ounce of shot and 3-inch shell with ¾ ounce of shot. The magnum shotgun shells are also made in 2¾- and 3-inch size. Although they are not necessarily bigger, they contain a heavier than standard load of shot: they contain about 20 per cent more shot than the standard shell.

Table 2-5.   Diameters of Wadding in Different Shotguns

Shotgun (gauge)	Diameter of Wadding (in inches)
8	0.845
10	0.784
12	0.738
16	0.671
20	0.623
28	0.557
0.410	0.415

Shotgun pellets have specific sizes and weights as shown in Table 2-3. Data on buckshot is given in Table 2-4. The size of a pellet is often difficult to measure after the shot is fired, because most of the pellets become deformed. However, the investigator can determine the shot size used by weighing the pellets after they are cleaned and dried. The standard shot chart (Fig. 2-12) will be of further help in determining the number or type of shot.

The measurements of *wads* may give some idea about the gauge of a shotgun (Table 2-5).

Rifled Shotgun Slugs.   Rifled slugs with spiral rifling (lands and grooves) on their surfaces are made for shotguns. In some hunting areas the rifles are illegal; that is why the hunters use slugs in their shotguns. The slugs are made of lead and are heavier at the nose than at the tail and are hollow at the base. They are available in 12, 16, 20, 28 and 0.410 gauges and can be loaded in shotguns with or without chokes. The spiral grooves on the slugs are meant to impart spinning effect to the slug, which is fired through the smooth bore of the shotgun, just the same way the rifling in a rifled firearm imparts spinning motion to the bullet. However, it is questionable whether in fact the slug spins or not when fired. Rifled slugs have good muzzle velocity and shooting with

Table 2-6.   Weights and Muzzle Velocities of Rifled Slugs

Gauge of Rifled Slugs	Weight (in ounces)	Muzzle Velocity (feet per second)
12	1	1600
16	7/8	1600
20	5/8	1600
28	1/2	1600
0.410	1/5	1800

them at moderate ranges is accurate. The slugs have much greater range than the pellets. Table 2-6 reflects the weights and muzzle velocities of various slugs.

REFERENCES

1. Camps, F. E. (ed.): Gradwohl's Legal Medicine. Bristol, John Wright & Sons, 1968.
2. Federal Bureau of Investigation: A Visual Aid for Firearms Identification. Washington, D.C.
3. Laycock, G: Barrels. *In* The Shotgunner's Bible. New York, Doubleday, 1969.
4. Riviere, B.: The Shotgun. *In* The Gunner's Bible. New York, Doubleday, 1973.
5. Sherrill, R.: The Saturday Night Special. New York, Charterhouse, 1973.

3

Forensic Ballistics

Forensic ballistics is conventionally known as firearms identification. However, in a real sense, ballistics should mean the study of the motion of a missile. This would include the study of the motion of the projectile within the firearm *(internal ballistics)*, the study of the motion of the projectile after it leaves the firearm *(external ballistics)* and the study of the effect of the projectile on a target *(terminal ballistics)*. In practice, modern ballistics laboratories and firearms experts are not only concerned with the identification of the gun, but they are also required to relate evidence ammunition to a certain gun by the study of markings on the bullets, cartridges and shells. They also render help in evaluating the distance of fire by conducting test fires.

The science of firearm identification is not very old; the first thoughts on firearm identification appeared in print in 1900.[3] In 1912, Professor Balthazard of Paris began his studies to identify the guns by examining fired bullets. He photographed various areas of two sets of fired bullets and compared the markings on enlarged photographs. Significant advances have since occurred in the field of forensic ballistics.

Bullets and empty cartridge cases are often found at the scene of a crime. Bullets may also be retrieved from the victim's body. In the investigation of a crime, positive identification of the firearm used in the crime is frequently essential to prove the guilt of the criminal. Often the success or failure of an investigation depends solely on the identification of the firearm. In view of the high incidence of firearm injuries and fatalities, one of the most common types of physical evidence that the criminalist is faced with is the gun and its ammunition. That is why the art and the science of identification of firearms is widely used in the investigation of a crime involving a gun and why many police departments are staffed with an expert who can assist in answering questions pertaining to forensic ballistics.

To answer the very important and frequently posed question, "Did this gun fire this ammunition?", the investigator must proceed systematically with the examination of (1) the gun; (2) the cartridge case; (3) the bullet; (4) the shotgun shell and (5) the pellets and wads.

EXAMINATION OF THE GUN

The gun used in a particular crime may or may not be found. If the gun is found in the possession of the suspect or elsewhere, the services of a firearm expert are needed to prove that the weapon in question was in fact the one that was used in the crime.

Proper documentation of all the details of examination of the gun used in a crime is important, for the examiner may be required to testify in court at a later date. The gun should first be photographed, and then the following information should be recorded:

1. Type of weapon: revolver, pistol, rifle or shotgun
2. Description of its condition
3. Length of the barrel
4. Manufacturer's marks and their locations
5. Serial number and its location
6. Description of the magazine, firing pin, breechlock and extractor or ejector
7. Rifling characteristics
8. Caliber or gauge of the weapon

Markings on Guns

Every modern gun manufactured in the United States is stamped with the manufacturer's name and address, the caliber and a serial number. Guns made in Europe bear "proof marks," and these marks can help determine the country of origin of the firearm. The serial number on the weapon is important because it can help identify the first owner and perhaps the criminal who used it; therefore, when a suspect weapon is received for examination a careful search for the serial number should be made. A general knowledge of where the serial numbers are placed in different guns can be useful. The work of Krcma (1961)[5] on the identification of pistols by serial numbers and that of Goddard (1934)[2] on proof marks should be consulted for such information.

If the serial number is not present on the gun, every effort should be made to restore the number. About 90 per cent of the serial numbers that have been removed can be restored. Mathews[6] has described a method for restoring numbers by using etching solutions. In the process of restoring serial numbers, it is important not to etch too rapidly.[9]

Sometimes helpful markings are not present on the gun, or if they are there, it may not be possible to restore them. Also, identification of guns made with imported parts, for example, the Saturday Night Specials, can be difficult. Great care should be exercised in examining such guns. A short discussion of the identification of some of the unusual handguns has been published by Smith.[7]

In recent years, surplus military rifles have entered the civilian market, and evidence of their increased use in crime is seen. The modern firearms examiner should be prepared to identify these weapons. Anderson and Krcma have detailed by diagrams breech faces of rifles and light machine guns from 17 countries and listed groove measurements on bullets fired by these weapons. The investigator faced with the question of identification of such weapons will find useful information in their article.

If the gun is not found at the scene of a crime, the investigator will have to proceed with other materials to draw conclusions about the weapon used. Such materials may consist of empty cartridge cases, bullets, shotgun shells, pellets and wads, clothing with bullet holes, gunshot wounds in the skin of the victim and photographs.

EXAMINATION OF THE BULLET

The identification of a firearm used in a crime often depends on the examination of the fired bullet. Therefore, an adequate amount of time should be spent in the examination of the evidence bullet. The investigation should consist of:

1. Visual inspection of the bullet
2. Recording of weight and diameter
3. Determination of caliber
4. Examination of marks on the bullet
5. Test firing

Visual Examination

The bullet should be cleansed with alcohol to remove extraneous materials such as blood, tissues, fibers, mud, grease, hair and particles of wood, glass, etc. All extraneous materials removed from the bullet should be retained if deemed important in the investigation. In many instances visual examination of the bullet helps decide the caliber of the bullet, especially if it is not deformed.

Weight and Diameter of Bullet

Each bullet should then be weighed with its fragments. If the bullet is intact, its weight may help determine its caliber. Table 3-1, giving weights of different bullets, will help in many cases. The bullets re-

Table 3-1. Determination of Caliber of a Fired Bullet
from its Weight

Weight (grains)	Type	Cartridge
15	Solid	.22 Short (gallery)
16–20	Solid	.22 BB Cap
27–30	Solid	.22 CB Cap
27–30	Solid	.22 Short
27–30	Solid	.22 Long
36–40	Solid	.22 Long Rifle
45	Jacketed	5.5 mm Velo Dog
48–51	Jacketed	.25 Auto
55	Jacketed	7 mm Nambu
70–77	Jacketed	.32 Auto.
70–77	Jacketed	.35 S & W Auto.
80–82	Solid	.32 Short R. F.
80–82	Solid	.32 Short Colt
80–82	Solid	.32 Long Colt
80–90	Solid	.320 Revolver
80–90	Solid	.320 Long Revolver
84–92	Jacketed	7.62 mm Tokarev
84–92	Jacketed	7.63 mm Mauser
85–88	Solid	.32 S & W
89–90	Solid	.32 Long R. F.
89–92	Solid	9 mm Parabellum, Iron
90–96	Jacketed	7.65 mm Parabellum
90–115	Solid and Jacketed	.32-20 W. C. F.
92–97	Jacketed	.380 Auto
97–101	Jacketed	9 mm Parabellum, Iron Core
98–100	Solid	.32 S & W Long
98–100	Solid	.32 Colt New Police
99–103	Jacketed	8 mm Nambu
110	Solid	.38 Special
113–127	Jacketed	9 mm Parabellum
114–118	Jacketed	9 mm Steyr
123–128	Jacketed	9 mm Mauser
125–130	Solid	.38 Short Colt
125–136	Jacketed	9 mm Bergmann Bayard
128–130	Jacketed	.38 Auto
145–150	Solid	.38 S & W
148–150	Solid	.38 Long Colt
148–150	Solid	.38 Colt New Police
148–150	Solid	.38 Special
158	Solid and Jacketed	.38 Special
158	Solid and Jacketed	.357 Magnum
160–167	Solid	.41 Short Colt
160–180	Solid and Jacketed	.38-40 W. C. F.
168–170	Solid	.44 Bulldog
173	Solid	.45 Auto
176–181	Jacketed	.380 Revolver MK. II
185	Jacketed	.45 Auto

(Table continued, overleaf)

Table 3-1.   Determination of Caliber of a Fired Bullet from its Weight (Continued)

Weight (grains)	Type	Cartridge
190–225	Solid	.44 S & W American
195–200	Solid	.41 Long Colt
200	Solid	.38 Special
200–217	Solid and Jacketed	.44-40 W. C. F.
200–230	Jacketed	.45. Auto.
210–222	Solid	.44 Colt
230	Solid	.45 Webley
230–255	Solid	.45 S & W
230–255	Solid	.45 Auto-Rim
240	Solid	.44 Magnum
246	Solid and Jacketed	.44 S & W Russian
246	Solid and Jacketed	.44 S & W Special
250–260	Solid	.45 Colt
265	Solid and Jacketed	.455 Revolver MK. II

(Courtesy of H. P. White Laboratory)

covered at the crime scenes and from the bodies of the victims are frequently damaged, and hence measurements of their diameters are difficult and often unreliable. Approximate diameters of intact and undeformed bullets are as follows:

0.22 caliber – $3/16$ inch
0.25 caliber – $1/4$ inch
0.32 caliber – $5/16$ inch
0.38 caliber – $3/8$ inch
0.45 caliber – $7/16$ inch

Markings on the Bullet

The most important markings on the bullets are those caused by the rifling of the gun. When the bullet travels through the barrel, rifling of the gun imparts repetitive marks on the surface of the bullet. In addition, marks caused by defects or irregularities in the barrel of the gun or in its muzzle may be found on fired bullets. On the other hand, in guns with constricted muzzles, rifling marks may be obliterated somewhat. Since no bullets are marked by the manufacturer for identification, any marks found on them are significant. The comparison of various marks on the evidence bullet with those on the test fired bullets often leads to the identification of the weapon.

Family characteristics of bullets can give clue to the make and model of the gun from which they were fired. These characteristics consist of:

Table 3-2.   Rifling Characteristics of Some Pistols and Revolvers

Gun	Number of Lands and Grooves	Direction of Twist	Pitch of Rifling (inches per turn)
Colt:			
0.22 Caliber, Sport Woodman	6	Left	14
Colt:			
0.32 Caliber, Colt Automatic	6	Left	16
Colt:			
0.38 Caliber, Official Police	6	Left	14
Harrington and Richardson:			
0.22 Caliber	6	Right	16
Iver Johnson:			
0.22 Caliber revolver	5	Right	15.75
0.32 Caliber revolver	5	Right	23.33
0.38 Caliber revolver	5	Right	23.33
Luger:			
7.65 mm Automatic	4	Right	9.84
9.0 mm Automatic	6	Right	9.84
Mauser: All models	6	Right	7.875
Remington:			
0.22 Rem. Automatic	6	Right	16
0.22 Short	5	Right	24
0.25 Rem. Automatic	6	Right	10
0.32 Rem. Automatic	7	Right	14
0.32 Rem. Auto. Pistol	7	Right	16
0.38 Rem.	6	Right	36
0.380 Rem. Auto. Pistol	7	Right	16
Smith and Wesson:			
0.22 Caliber	6	Right	10 or 15
0.32 A. C. P. Auto.	6	Right	12
0.38 and 0.38/44 Special	5	Right	18.75
0.45 S & W Schofield Model			
Revolver	5	Right	24
Sturm, Ruger:			
0.22 Standard Auto.	6	Right	14
Webley and Scott			
0.22 Pistols and revolvers	7	Right	15
0.25 Auto. Pistol	6	Right	10
0.32 Mark IV Pocket Revolver	7	Right	15
0.32 Auto. Pistol	6	Right	10

(Table continued, overleaf)

Table 3-2.   Rifling Characteristics of Some Pistols and Revolvers (Continued)

Gun	Number of Lands and Grooves	Direction of Twist	Pitch of Rifling (inches per turn)
0.38 Mark IV Pocket Revolver	7	Right	15
0.38 Auto. Pistol	6	Right	10
0.38 Gov't. Mark IV Revolver	7	Right	18
0.455 Auto. Pistol	6	Right	10
0.455 Mark I–VI Revolver	7	Right	20

(Information derived from Kirk, P. L.: Crime Investigation. New York, Interscience Publishers, 1953; and Mathews, J. H.: Firearm Identification, volume 1. Springfield, Charles C Thomas, 1973.)

1. Number of lands and grooves. In most of the handguns manufactured in the United States, the number of lands and grooves are five or six. Four-groove rifling is less common. No guns are now made with three grooves. The majority of the firearms used in the commission of crime nowadays are rifled with four, five or six grooves with a right-hand twist or six grooves with a left-hand twist.

2. Direction of twist of rifling. The direction of rifling twist can help exclude certain families of guns. For instance, bullets fired from the "Colt type" guns have grooves slanting to the left and those from the "Smith & Wesson type" have grooves slanting to the right. The Colt Company is the only manufacturer in the United States producing a left-hand twist. A short listing of the rifling characteristics—direction of twist, number of grooves and pitch of rifling of some of the guns—is given in Table 3-2.

3. Width of lands and grooves. The widths of lands and grooves vary in different guns. In some guns the width of the grooves is the same as the width of the lands while in others the lands are wider or narrower than the grooves. The lands in the barrel of the gun cause grooves on the bullet. The measurements of these grooves will give some idea about the width of the lands of the gun (Table 3-3).

4. Depth of grooves. It is difficult to measure the depths of the grooves on the bullets, and even if the measurements are possible, they are rarely useful in establishing the identity of the weapon.

The caliber, the number of lands and grooves and the direction of rifling twist are the most useful criteria in the examination of a bullet.

Table 3-3.   Determination of Caliber of Fired Bullet
From Rifling Widths

Land width plus groove width (inches)	Caliber indicated	No. of grooves
.094–.101	.22, 5.5 mm, 5.6 mm	7
.109–.118	.22, 5.5 mm, 5.6 mm	6
.127–.132	.25, 6.35 mm	6
.131–.142	.22, 5.5 mm, 5.6 mm	5
.134–.141	.30, .32, 7.65 mm	7
.152–.158	.25, 6.35 mm	5
.154–.163	.35, .357, 38, 9 mm	7
.157–.165	.30, .32, 7.65 mm	6
.162–.169	.35 S & W. Auto.	6
.164–.177	.22, 5.5 mm, 5.6 mm	4
.180–.190	.35, .357, 38, 9 mm	6
.188–.198	.30, .32, 7.65 mm	5
.190–.197	.25, 6.35 mm	4
.197–.207	.45, .455	7
.201–.210	.38/40, .41	6
.216–.228	.35, .357, .38, 9 mm	5
.218–.225	.44	6
.230–.242	.45, .455	6
.235–.247	.30, .32, 7.65 mm	4
.242–.252	.38/48, .41	5
.262–.270	.44	5
.270–.285	.35, .357, .38, 9 mm	4
.276–.290	.45, .455	5
.302–.315	.38/40, .41	4
.327–.338	.44	4
.345–.363	.45, .455	4

(Courtesy of B. D. Munhall, H. P. White Laboratory).

Examination of Jacketed Bullets

Many of the bullets used in automatic pistols, rifles and machine guns are jacketed. The jacket is made of copper or cupro-nickel. The "soft nosed" bullets used for hunting and the "hollow point" bullets are almost completely covered with the jacket. Therefore, when such bullets are used, jackets of the bullets form important pieces of evidence, and careful examination of the jackets or fragments of jackets should be made for rifling marks or other identifying markings.

Test Firing

This is done for various reasons. The manufacturer test fires the gun to check its operation and safety after the gun is made. Test fires are also

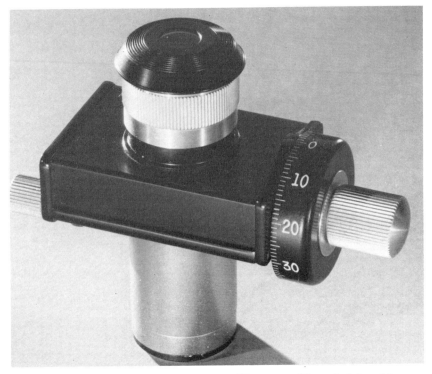

Fig. 3-1.   Filar micrometer eyepiece (Courtesy of Bausch & Lomb).

done for investigative purposes to determine the range of fire and also to recover test-fired bullets for comparison of marks on the test-fired bullet and the evidence bullet.

For the purpose of obtaining fired bullets for the study of markings on them, it is most advisable to obtain ammunition similar to the kind used in the commission of crime. If any unspent ammunition is found in the suspect gun, it should be used for test fires. Weapons in good condition generally produce bullets that are easy to match.

Test fires for the recovery of bullets may be done in different ways. Shots may be fired into cotton batting or oiled sawdust. Some workers use blocks of ice to shoot into; bullets shot into ice show good markings with no artefactual deformations. However, this is not a practical approach. Many institutions use water tanks, which may be vertical or horizontal with a system to recover fired bullets.

Sutherland and Krcma[8] have described test bullet recovery methods. They recommend various forms of boxes and tanks for military and sporting rifles and water tanks for all handguns, low power rifles and submachine guns.

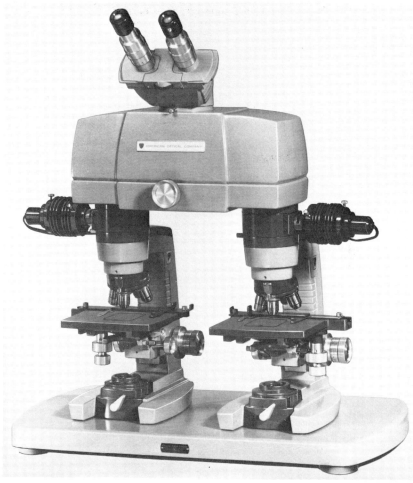

Fig. 3-2.   Comparison microscope (Courtesy of American Optical Corporation).

Methods of comparison of bullets have changed with times. In the early years of the 20th century, comparison of bullets was done by photographing areas on fired bullets and comparing them with those on the evidence bullet. Then came the development of filar micrometer (Fig. 3-1), a small tool that facilitated measurement of widths of grooves on test fired bullets and evidence bullet for comparison. Comparison of marks nowadays is made with comparison microscopes (Fig. 3-2, 3-3) or comparison camera (Fig. 3-4). *The comparison microscope* consists of two compound microscopes which allow comparison of two objects by look-

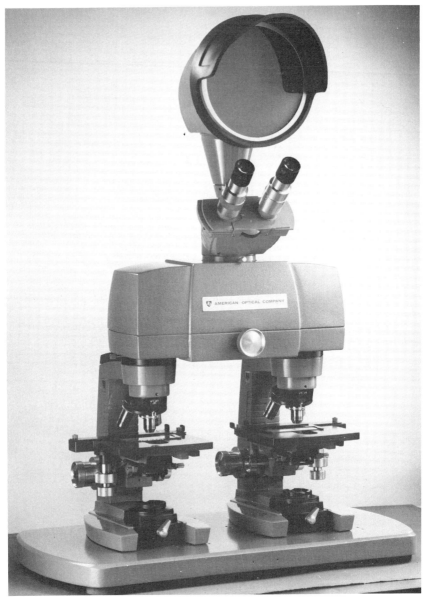

Fig. 3-3. Comparison microscope (Courtesy of American Optical Corporation).

ing through a single eyepiece. The single field allows examination of one object in one half of the field and another object in the other half of the field (Fig. 3-5). This microscope is very useful for comparing markings on the bullets and cartridges. *The comparison camera* allows com-

Fig. 3-4. Comparison camera (Courtesy of American Optical Corporation).

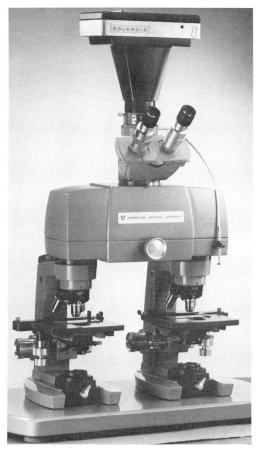

parison of two objects just the same way as the comparison microscope, but it does so by giving large images on a ground-glass screen making the comparison easy and less strenuous to the eye. In addition, one can photograph the images on the screen.

CARTRIDGE IDENTIFICATION

As on the bullet, there may be important repetitive markings on the cartridge case that can help determine the type and make of the gun used in a crime. Although the work on cartridges is not as rewarding as the work on bullets, cartridge cases may at times contribute to the solution of a crime. The comparison of marks on the evidence cartridge case and the test-fired cartridge case may lead to the identification of

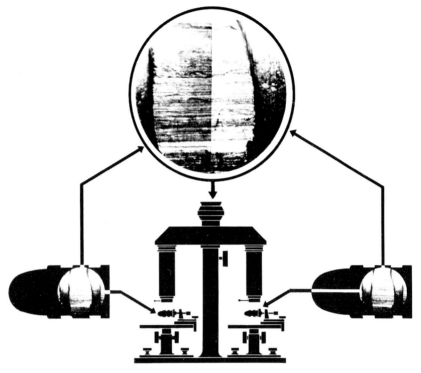

Fig. 3-5.   A diagram illustrating the principle of the comparison microscope in the examination of markings on bullets (Illustration by B. D. Munhall. Courtesy of the Institute of Applied Science, Chicago).

the gun. For test fires, as far as possible, unspent cartridges in the suspect weapon should be used. If these are not available, cartridges similar to the one suspected to have been fired should be used. Several shots should be fired to obtain multiple cartridge cases.

Fired cartridge cases bear two sets of markings: those imprinted by the manufacturer and those caused in the process of firing. Recently manufactured cartridges and shells bear symbols and letters of identification; this is useful because modern ammunition is used in over 95 per cent of crimes committed with firearms. Pistol cartridges are stamped with manufacturer's mark and the size of the cartridge.

Initial examination of the evidence cartridge case should include notations about the general features of the cartridge such as shape (rimmed, rimless, straight, tapered or necked), caliber (usually stamped in centerfire cases), composition (brass, nickel-plated, copper, plated steel or paper) and manufacturer's name, trademark or initial.

Comparison of the cases of evidence and of fired cartridge cases can

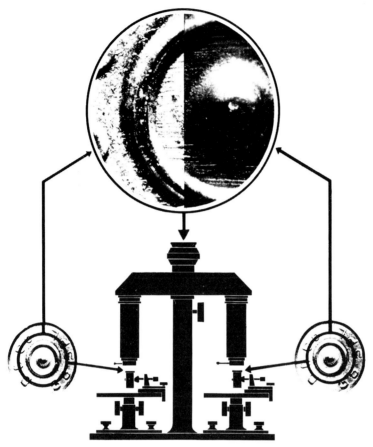

Fig. 3-6. The use of a comparison microscope in the examination of cartridges (Illustration by B. D. Munhall. Courtesy of Institute of Applied Science, Chicago).

be simply done with the help of a magnifying glass. However, for positive identification of various marks on the cartridge cases, more careful examination of the evidence and test-fired cases should be made with either a stereoscopic microscope or a comparison microscope (Fig. 3-6). Enlarged photographs of the cases and the markings of them make good visual evidence in the court.

The marks that may be present on the cartridge cases caused in the process of firing are (1) firing pin marks; (2) breechlock marks, (3) magazine marks; (4) extractor marks and (5) ejector marks. The size, shape and location of these marks should be noted. If marks identical to the ones on the evidence cartridge cases are reproduced on the test fire ammunition the identity of the gun in question is established. A few comments on various marks follow.

Firing Pin Marks

The firing pin is a device used to cause the shell to fire. When the pin strikes the shell, it makes an impression of the striking portion of the firing pin on the shell. Such firing pin impressions are the most distinguishing of the marks and often have characteristic features that can exclude a certain gun or suggest certain makes of guns. The shapes of the rimfire firing pin impressions as classified by the H. P. White Laboratory in Bel Air, Maryland are bar, rectangular, round, semicircular, and special. Another classification suggested by Mathews[4] subdivides firing pin impressions into bar, rectangular (square), rectangular (narrow), rectangular (broad), round (large), round (small), semicircular (large), semicircular (small), and special. The centerfire firing pin marks also have individuality and can be matched. The firing pin ends may be tapering, rounded, blunt or flat and leave markings that correspond to the contour of the ends.

The firing pin impressions are not always well defined, and in fact, the same pin may produce variable impressions, while firing pins of weapons of different makes may make similar impressions. Therefore, it is important to fire multiple shots for comparison of firing pin marks.

Breechlock Marks

These markings are caused by the impact of the head of the shell against the breechlock. The breechlock markings are distinct, and it is easy to compare such marks on different shells fired from the same gun.

Magazine Marks

In automatic weapons, scratches are caused on the cartridge or shell during loading due to friction with the metallic parts of the magazine. Sometimes these marks are distinct, but other times they are not. Because of the variability in the marks, they are rarely useful in positively identifying the weapon.

Extractor Marks

The marks caused by the extractor on a shell are important because their presence would readily exclude all pistols that do not have extractors. The extractor marks are not only useful in determining the type of gun, but they also give clues as to the position of the shell in the chamber of the gun at the time of firing. When the suspect in a crime disclaims ownership of the gun or in "no gun" cases, the extractor marks are important. These marks are found on the forward face of the shell rim. It must be remembered that some guns with loose extractors may not give good extractor marks.

Ejector Marks

The pistols that are fitted with special ejectors cause ejector marks on the head of the shell. The majority of the modern pistols have special ejectors. The ejector marks are not as important as extractor marks, because they show great variability. Some ejector marks on the shells are well-defined, whereas the others are almost unidentifiable. Also, some pistols equipped with special ejectors do not cause any mark at all. Nevertheless, the presence of an ejector mark would, in most cases, help distinguish a gun with an ejector from the one without an ejector.

In recent years, scanning electron microscopy has been applied to study the markings on bullets and cartridge cases. The articles describing the work are reviewed in Chapter 17.

SPECTROGRAPHIC ANALYSIS

Sometimes it may be necessary to do spectrographic analysis to establish the composition of a cartridge case, a bullet or fragments thereof. Spectrographic analysis depends on the emission of light by metals heated to a high temperature; from the wavelengths in the spectrum the metals in the material can be identified. By this investigation it may be possible to compare the spent ammunition used in the crime with the unspent ammunition found on the suspect.

REFERENCES

1. Anderson, E. J. and Krcma, V.: Military rifle and light machine gun identification notes. J. For. Sci., *10*:294, 1965.
2. Goddard, C. H.: Proof Tests and Proof Marks. Army Ordnance Nov–Dec. 1933, Jan–Feb. 1934, March–April, 1934, May–June, 1934. July–Aug. 1934.
3. Hatcher, J. S., Jury, F. J. and Weller, J.: The History of Firearms Identification. *In* Samworth, T. G. (ed.): Firearms Investigation Identification and Evidence. Harrisburg, Stackpole, 1957.
4. Kirk, P. L.: Crime Investigation. New York, Interscience Publishers, 1953.
5. Krcma, V.: The identification of pistols by serial numbers and other markings. J. For. Sci., *6*:479, 1961.
6. Mathews, J. H.: Firearm Identification, volume 1. Springfield, Charles C Thomas, 1973.
7. Smith, L. L.: Unusual handguns—Unlawfully possessed or used in crime. J. For. Sci., *6*:501, 1961.
8. Sutherland, W. W. and Krcma, V.: Test bullet recovery. J. For. Sci., *7*:493, 1962.
9. Turner, R. F.: Forensic Science and Laboratory Technics. Springfield, Charles C Thomas, 1949.

4

The Scene Investigation of
a Nonfatal Shooting

In any medicolegal investigation of a nonfatal shooting incident, the most important question to be answered is whether the shooting was accidental, self-inflicted with suicidal intent or a criminal assault.

In the majority of cases, the manner of injury is quite obvious. Accidental shooting is frequently explained by the witnesses or else the findings at the scene of injury suggest an accident. Suicidal shootings are also frequently associated with many clues. In cases in which the accidental or suicidal nature of the injury is obvious, no extraordinary measures of investigation are necessary. There are, however, some cases in which the manner of shooting is not clear and others in which the shooting is distinctly criminal. These cases require meticulous investigation. In this chapter, details of the line of investigation to be followed in such cases are discussed.

THE FIRST CALL

The police officer is most likely to be the first one to be informed about a shooting incident. When a call is received, and it appears that the shooting is criminal, a team of investigators should respond to the call. Investigation of a crime is teamwork and, as far as possible, no one person should attempt to handle the responsibility singlehanded. Every investigator should be prepared with plans and equipment to conduct an investigation. If the call reveals that the victim is alive, an ambulance equipped for emergency care should be ordered to the scene, if this has not already been done. The documentation of the investigation should begin with the notation of time of receiving the first call.

THE SCENE OF THE SHOOTING

On arrival at the scene of the shooting, if the investigators find the victim alive, all their actions must be directed toward securing medical care for the victim. After receiving whatever help can be given at the scene, the patient should be rushed to the hospital. If the condition of the victim permits, questions about the circumstances of the shooting should be asked and the victim's answers noted immediately.

One of the first steps of a medicolegal investigation at the scene of a crime should be documentation by description, diagrams and photographs of the locations of the victim and all the materials of evidence. Therefore, a general survey of the scene should be made to establish the location of items of evidence. If the victim has to be moved, a sketch representing the location and posture of the victim should be marked at the scene with chalk or ink marker. One investigator should accompany the patient to the hospital for furtherance of the investigation.

After the important aspects of the treatment of the victim are attended to, the law enforcement agents in charge of medicolegal investigation at the scene of shooting should proceed to gather information and evidence. The investigation should consist of:

1. Questioning of witnesses and interrogation of suspect
2. Photographs of the scene
3. Search for fingerprints
4. Collection of items of evidence

Questioning of Witnesses and Interrogation of Suspect

Interrogation of the witnesses is very important in criminal cases. Proper questioning of the witnesses can lead to solution of the crime. According to Mulbar the basis for the solution of 99 per cent of all cases is furnished by proper questioning.[3] The interrogation of the witnesses at the scene of crime is especially significant, because the witnesses have the facts fresh in their minds and would be able to describe accurately what they heard or saw. The time factor is significant. For instance, if the shooting is witnessed shortly before the arrival of the investigator, vivid description of events, with time sequence, will be spontaneously forthcoming from the witnesses.

Interrogation of the suspect is a very sensitive part of the investigation. There must be a very calculated and careful approach in this direction; the task of interrogating the suspect requires patience and considerable effort. Many works describing the art of interrogation are available and the police investigator must familiarize himself with the techniques.[2,3] It must be emphasized that the suspect must be informed of his rights before he is asked to make statements of any kind.

Photographs of the Scene

The importance of photography as an aid in criminal investigation cannot be overemphasized. Before and after any items of evidence are moved, photographs must be made from different angles to document respective positions of various items of evidence, including the position of the victim. Details of various aspects of this investigation are discussed in Chapter 7.

Search for Fingerprints

At the scene of the shooting, careful consideration must be given to the aspect of fingerprints on various objects. The investigator should always ask himself a question: Am I going to disturb or destroy any evidence of value if I touch or move anything? This is important because an article may be picked up carelessly, resulting in obliteration of valuable fingerprints on it, or new prints may be added to some articles at the same time erasing the suspect's prints. All areas likely to bear suspect's fingerprints, especially door knobs, glassware, and the gun, must be processed for fingerprints before they are touched or moved. Only after this work of processing the fingerprints on various articles is completed should the process of collecting evidence begin.

Collection of Evidence

The essentials of a good investigation consist of the knowledge of what evidence should be collected and the knowledge of how best to preserve the collected evidence and process it for the desired purpose.

Some of the important principles to be kept in mind are: (1) Every article even remotely likely to be helpful in the investigation must be collected after the relative location of each article is documented. It is advisable to collect more than is needed rather than less. Failure to collect some of the evidence could result in miscarriage of justice. (2) Every small or large item should be placed in a separate container. (3) Every article collected must bear identifying marks. (4) Any item even remotely likely to carry fingerprints must be processed for prints before it is moved or touched.

The investigator at a scene of crime must always be equipped with containers and labels. In the cases of shooting, the physical evidence that is likely to be of importance will be found:

1. On the victim's body

2. On the suspect's body
3. At the scene of crime

Collection of Evidence from the Victim's Body. In a nonfatal shooting case there is usually very little opportunity to collect materials of evidential value from the victim's body at the scene of crime, because it is necessary to rush the victim to the hospital as fast as possible. If, however, there is opportunity to collect such evidence, the articles of importance may be the victim's clothes, hair or fibers on the body, blood spots on the clothes or body and sometimes gunpowder residues.

Whenever possible all *clothes* of evidential value, especially those showing bullet holes, should be removed from the victim before he is taken to the hospital. As far as possible, cutting of the clothes should be avoided, particularly in the area of the bullet holes. The clothes should be placed in separate labelled containers. If they are wet, they should be dried, not washed, and folded in such a way that the areas of bullet holes and gunpowder soiling are not disturbed or contaminated.

All extraneous *hairs and fibers* on the victim's body should be collected and kept in separate clean containers. It may later be necessary to compare the hair on the victim's body with the suspect's hair. In addition to the extraneous hair on the victim's body, a few hairs of the victim should also be retained for comparison with the extraneous hair. Fibers of clothing may have been left on the victim from the suspect's clothing. These could be important and should be carefully collected. Particular attention should be paid to the presence of such fibers, hairs, and other items of trace evidence in the fingernails of the victim, especially in cases of a struggle.

If the Victim Goes to the Hospital. If the victim is sent to the hospital for treatment of the gunshot wounds, some evidence will go with the victim. Duties of the investigator accompanying the victim to the hospital and of the doctor rendering treatment, concerning the preservation of evidence on the victim's body are outlined below:

Duties of the Police Investigator. The investigator, who accompanies the patient to the hospital, has the primary responsibility of collecting and preserving the evidence that goes to the hospital with the victim. The investigating police officer should inform the hospital staff about the circumstances of the shooting and explain the significance of the materials of evidence on or in the victim's body.

Such evidence would consist of (1) bullet holes in the clothes if they had not been removed at the scene of the shooting; (2) bullets in the victim's body; (3) gunpowder on the victim's hands; (4) trace evidence—hairs, fibers; and (5) victim's blood. Even at the expense of being criticized for being overzealous, the police officer should, as gently and tactfully as possible, make the hospital staff appreciate the importance of their cooperation. They should be requested to help preserve evidence.

The attending staff should be told not to cut the clothing, as far as possible, through the bullet holes. As soon as the clothes bearing bullet holes are removed from the victim's body, the police officer should take charge of them. Any loose objects falling from the victim's clothes, especially loose bullets or other items of spent ammunition must, of course, be carefully preserved.

The surgeon may be requested to describe the external gunshot wounds carefully, for medicolegal purposes, before they are excised or extended. Photographic documentation is most advisable before the skin wounds are excised. If the wounds are excised, an examination of the excised tissue with a view to estimate the distance and the angle of fire should be sought. The surgeon may remove bullets, pellets or wads from the body. The police officer should obtain these from the surgeon for ballistic work.

Blood typing of the victim's blood may be necessary, in some instances, for comparison with the blood groups of blood spots that may be found on the suspect. Therefore, a request should be made to obtain the victim's blood from the hospital. Other items that could not be collected from the victim's body at the scene of the shooting may be collected when he is in the hospital.

With respect to any materials of evidential value in the investigation of a crime, the chain of custody is important. Therefore, every time an item of evidence passes from one person to another such a fact should be recorded and a receipt issued. The police officer obtaining the evidence from the hospital should give receipts indicating the description of the items, the date, time and place and the names of the parties giving and receiving the articles.

All statements made by the patient during the course of the hospital stay should be carefully recorded, particularly in criminal cases. If the patient is likely to die, arrangements should be made to obtain a valid dying declaration.

Duties of the Doctor.   In the case of a nonfatal shooting, the police may accompany the victim to the hospital. If the police have not already been informed, the hospital or the treating physician should report the case to them as soon as possible.

The hospital records may be summoned to court at a later date; therefore, maintenance of proper records is important. The date and time of admission and all the available details of the circumstances of the shooting must be accurately recorded. It is most advisable to record the exact statements of the victim and of the witnesses accompanying the victim. It is also important to describe in detail the nature and positions of the gunshot wounds as well as note the treatment and progress.

Whenever possible, the gunshot wounds should be photographed in their original state and these photographs should be retained as part of the patient's records. The photographs should bear proper identification marks.

X-rays are invaluable in determining the location of the bullets in the body. Whenever X-rays are made, they should bear proper identification marks, and they should be preserved with the hospital records.

It may be necessary to perform surgery on a patient with firearm injuries. No doubt the welfare of the patient should be of paramount concern to the treating physician, but it is also important to bear in mind the medicolegal aspects of the case. Therefore, if surgery is to be performed it is advisable to preserve, if at all possible, the gunshot wounds in their original state. If the wound needs to be excised or extended, it is especially important to photograph and describe it. If surgical exploration is performed, notes should be made about the direction of the bullet track within the body. These records will be valuable to the surgeon when he is summoned to testify at a later date. All excised tissue, particularly the wounds in the skin or the fragments of bone shattered by bullet, must be retained. Failure to do so can result in a miscarriage of justice as illustrated by the following case.

A 40-year-old man was 20 feet from a man to his right and 10 feet from another man to his left. The man on the right fired three shots from his 0.38 caliber gun in an attempt to shoot the man on the left. The man on the left returned fire once with a 0.32 caliber revolver. The man in the middle, an innocent bystander, was the only one who sustained gunshot wounds. He was taken to the hospital. In the hospital the neurosurgeon noted a gunshot wound in the right forehead region and another in the left forehead region but did not describe or photograph the wounds. For exploratory surgery, he made a horizontal incision across the forehead through both gunshot wounds. He also excised the wounds to debride the skin and discarded the tissue. Multiple fractures of the frontal bone on both sides were seen with severe lacerations and contusions of the frontal lobes of the brain. The surgeon removed many of the fragments of the bone and discarded them. The man remained unconscious and died two days later.

At autopsy it was not possible to localize the positions of the gunshot wounds or to determine whether they were entrance or exit wounds because the skin wounds and large portions of comminuted frontal bone had been removed by the surgeon and no descriptions were made. A portion of a bullet was found lodged in the left temporal bone. This was so deformed and damaged that it was not possible to determine as to which of the two guns in question had fired it.

The loss of evidence was a principal reason for failure in getting conviction of either of the two men involved in the shooting.

The surgeon may remove a bullet or bullets from the victim's body. Such bullets may bear valuable rifling marks on them. In order to preserve these marks, the bullets so removed should be handled as little as possible with clamps or forceps. When removed they should be placed in envelopes or cardboard boxes wrapped in soft paper or cotton. Each container should be labelled with such information as the name of the patient, location in the body from where the bullet was removed, name of the surgeon removing the bullet and the date of removal. It is a common practice to send these bullets to the pathology laboratory. The pathologist may discard such items with other specimens during routine periodical clearances. In order to prevent such a mishap's resulting in the loss of important medicolegal evidence, it is best to deliver the bullets removed from the victim of firearm injuries to the police.

Receipts must be obtained from the police whenever such items as clothes, excised gunshot wounds and bullets (or pellets and wads) removed from the victim's body are delivered to them.

Collection of Evidence from the Suspect's Body.   If a person is in custody, with reason for believing him to be the assailant, all care should be expended to collect evidence from him and preserve it. In cases of fatal or nonfatal shooting, a suspect is likely to be at the scene of the crime if he is promptly arrested prior to escape, if he decides to admit to the shooting or if he has made up his mind to present the shooting incident as an accident or as an act of self defense. Whenever a suspect is apprehended, the materials of useful evidence that are present on his body will consist of:

1. Clothes with trace evidence
2. Victim's hair, clothing fibers and blood spots
3. Gunpowder and other evidence on the hands
4. Gun used in the crime
5. Unspent ammunition and empty cartridges or shells

The suspect's clothes may be useful in the investigation in various ways. The pockets of the clothing may contain identification papers, ammunition, etc. On the clothing there may be trace evidence such as victim's hair, clothing fibers and blood. The suspect's gun may be in his hands or in his pockets. The suspect's hands may reveal the presence of gunpowder, and in cases of a struggle there may be trace evidence in the suspect's fingernails. In addition to trace evidence on the suspect's body and clothing, it is important to retain the suspect's hair and blood so that comparisons can be made when necessary. As with any other evidence, every item taken from the suspect's body should be recorded, placed in a separate container and properly labelled.

Collection of Evidence from the Scene of Shooting.   The scene of a criminal shooting may yield many valuable pieces of evidence. It should be emphasized again that only after a general survey of the scene is made, photographs taken and fingerprints processed, should the actual collection of evidence begin. The items of importance that should be looked for are

1. The gun
2. Fired bullets
3. Empty cartridge cases, shells and wads
4. Hairs, fibers and blood spots

5. Objects struck by or containing spent bullets—wood, cement, etc.
6. Glass shattered by bullets
7. Areas showing fingerprints and footprints

At the scene of an accidental shooting the gun is invariably present, unless it is stolen or inadvertently removed. At the locations of suicidal shootings the gun is also usually present. If the gun is missing, this could arouse suspicions of foul play. Sometimes the relatives of the victim move the weapon to conceal suicide. Occasionally the gun is stolen, especially if the victim is in an open area.

In most cases of criminal shooting, the gun is not found at the scene of the shooting. Through error the criminal may leave the gun behind. He may place the weapon in the victim's hand to mislead the investigators. If the gun is found at the scene of the shooting, the significance of its presence there must be properly evaluated.

Bullets that go through the body of the victim or ones that do not hit the victim will be present at the scene of the shooting. Those fired bullets should be carefully searched for at the scene of the shooting. The fired bullets may be found either loose or embedded in the walls, ceiling or furniture. If the bullet has penetrated any object, every effort must be made to retrieve it, and while doing so, care should be exercised not to damage it. If the shot has passed through glass, fragments of glass should be collected. The examination of these pieces may help determine the direction of fire.[1] Even small fragments of a bullet may bear useful rifling marks. If a shotgun is used, there may be pellets or wads at the scene. The bullets, fragments or pellets could lead to the identification of the firearm used in the crime and ultimately to the solution of the case.

Empty cartridge cases, shells and wads found at the scene of the shooting can be important. Their positions may help determine the direction of fire. The examination of the cartridge cases and shells, as described in Chapter 3, may disclose markings that could relate these to the firing gun. The size and composition of the wadding may give some information about the type of ammunition and the gauge of the shotgun. Other trace evidence such as hairs, fibers and blood should be collected from the scene of the shooting in just the same way as from the victim and the suspect. In some instances, in addition to fingerprints, foot and footwear prints may be found at the scene. These should be examined carefully for possible clues.

HANDLING AND TRANSMITTAL OF EVIDENCE

Proper handling of the evidence already gathered is as important as any other aspect of the investigation. It may be necessary to send the articles of evidence to laboratories for examination.

If the materials of evidential value are to be transmitted to the FBI laboratory, the advice outlined by the FBI in their publication *Suggestions for Handling of Physical Evidence* should be followed. They suggest that the firearms should be identified with an attached string tag on which the name of the weapon, its caliber and serial number together with the date of finding the weapon and the name of the sender should appear. It should be unloaded first and then wrapped in paper and placed in a cardboard or wooden box. It could be sent by registered mail or Railway Express or air express. The bullets (not cartridges) should be identified with initials on the base, cartridges with initials on the outside of the case near bullet end and cartridge cases (shells) with initials preferably on the inside near the open end or on the outside near the open end. Each of these items should be wrapped with cotton or soft paper and placed in separate pill, match or powder boxes in such a way that they do not shift within the container during transit. The bullets and cartridge cases should be sent by registered mail, but the cartridge and other ammunition should be sent by Railway Express only. Paraffin for gunpowder tests must be placed in containers free of any nitrate-containing substances after it is wrapped in waxed paper or sandwich bag and padded all around with cotton to prevent shifting within the container. To prevent any damage to the configuration of the paraffin, the container holding it should be placed in a larger box with absorbent material. The container should be appropriately identified with a label on its outside and sent by registered mail. The clothing to be examined for gunpowder should be dried if wet and placed flat between layers of paper. Then it should be wrapped to prevent shaking so that no residue will be transferred or lost. It is advisable to send a letter under separate cover about the evidence being sent.

REFERENCES

1. Federal Bureau of Investigation: Handbook of Forensic Science. Washington, D.C., U.S. Government Printing Office, 1974.
2. Inbau, F. E. and Reid, J. E.: Lie Detection and Criminal Interrogation. ed. 3. Baltimore, Williams and Wilkins, 1953.
3. Mulbar, H.: Interrogation. Springfield, Charles C Thomas, 1951.

5

The Scene Investigation
of a Firearm Fatality

The scene investigation is of paramount importance in any medicolegal inquiry into a death. The visit to a scene of death crystalizes the circumstances surrounding it and adds substantially to the total knowledge of the case. Furthermore, an on-the-spot study of the circumstances of death prompts one to look for things that would not ordinarily come to mind if the scene were not visited.

The police investigators, with a ballistics expert and a medical investigator, should form a team to investigate a firearm fatality. Together they can answer most of the questions pertaining to a death from gunshot wounds. As in any other medicolegal investigation of death, the study of a case of gunshot wound should aim at answering the principal questions concerning the cause and the manner of death, the time of death and the identification of the deceased. There are also other questions involved in the case of gunshot wounds, such as:

1. Were the injuries caused by gunfire?
2. Which one of the wounds was fatal?
3. What was the course of the projectile in the body?
4. How long could the victim have survived after being shot?
5. How much activity could the victim have performed after the shooting?
6. Was death solely due to firearm injuries?
7. How many shots were fired? How many hit the victim?
8. What was the range of fire?
9. What was the angle of fire?
10. What was the position of the victim when shot?
11. What was the position of the shooter in relation to the victim?
12. What was the make, model, caliber, type of action and serial number of the gun?
13. Did a particular gun fire one or more shots?

14. Was the firearm in proper functioning or operating condition?
15. Could the firearm have accidentally discharged?
16. Is the fired bullet, cartridge case or shot consistent with the gun?
17. If there are multiple wounds, entrance and exit wounds, could they have been produced by one bullet?
18. If multiple bullets are involved, were they fired from one or more guns?

In presenting such questions, a systematic evaluation of a case of gunshot wounds is suggested with the following points in mind:

1. Preservation and collection of evidence at the scene of death
2. Identification of the weapon
3. Discovery of the wounds and identification of gunshot wounds
4. Number and location of wounds in the clothing and on the body
5. Features of gunshot wounds and adjacent areas
6. Range of fire (contact, close, distant)
7. Angle of fire
8. Number of shots fired
9. Course of the projectile in the body
10. Retrieval of the bullet or pellets and determination of the type of gun
11. Retrieval of foreign materials (fabric, wadding and so on) from the wound track in the body
12. Period of survival
13. Degree of volitional activity after shooting
14. Identification of lethal wound
15. Recording of injuries for presentation in courts (reports, diagrams, photographs, x-rays)
16. Special investigations (fingerprints, blood type, toxicologic studies, histologic examinations, test firing, identification of gunpowder residue, and so on)

The facets of investigation that can help the police officers and the medical investigator accumulate all pertinent information are the examination of the scene of death, of the body and of the weapon and the ancillary investigations. At the scene of death, the team of investigators should be concerned with the following specific aims:

1. Study of the circumstances of shooting
2. Preservation of evidence
3. Examination of the body, the gun and the spent and unspent ammunition
4. Collection of evidence
5. Recording of findings
6. Preliminary decisions on the line of further investigation

The investigation must be a cooperative effort designed to achieve the ultimate goals of the inquiry. Therefore, the tasks of the police officers and the medical investigator should be mutually complementary. No precise line can be drawn to separate the functions of various investigators, since all parties may be involved in certain aspects of the investigation. However, an attempt is made here to discuss in broad terms the roles of the police and the medical investigator at the scene of death.

ROLE OF THE POLICE INVESTIGATOR

When a death is reported by telephone, whether by a relative of the decedent, a funeral director or just a passerby or a witness to the death, the police officer should report to the scene and summon the Coroner or Medical Examiner. At the scene of death his principal functions include those mentioned above. Some details on these aspects of the investigation are discussed in the preceding chapter. The reader, therefore, is advised to refer to those details to get a complete picture of the police investigator's functions.

Circumstances of the Shooting

An important aspect of a shooting death is the determination of the manner of death. In a majority of the cases, the circumstances of death become obvious at the beginning of the *conversation with the witnesses* and the manner of death becomes clear. The *location of the shooting* (hunting area, locked room, entertainment spot) may give a ready clue to the manner of death. The presence or absence of the gun at the scene of death is an important factor. If the gun is present, suicide or accident is more likely; its absence should arouse suspicion of foul play. The possibility of alteration of the scene should always be kept in mind. The *type of gun* that caused death and its condition may sometimes help draw conclusions about the manner of death. If suicide is thought to be a possibility, the personal history of the decedent can clinch the issue.

Preservation of Evidence

It must be stressed again that before the examination of any scene of death is commenced, due consideration should be given to the aspect of preservation of evidence. If a crime is committed, the detection of fingerprints on the weapon (if present at the scene), on doorknobs and so on may solve the murder. Therefore, every care should be taken, as has already been stressed in the preceding chapter, to preserve such evidence.

First of all, photographs of the scene, the body and the gun should be taken before anything is touched. The gun may then be picked up for examination by holding it near the muzzle with gloved hands.

Another important precaution to be taken at the scene concerns the handling of the clothes and the body. If there is gunpowder residue on the victim's hands, it should be preserved by wrapping the hands in dry, clean plastic bags. For detailed examination in the autopsy room, the clothes should preferably be left on the body undisturbed. Specific instructions should be given to the funeral director who is going to move the body to the necropsy room not to unclothe it and especially not to embalm it.

Collection of Evidence

Details about various articles of evidential value that should be collected are presented in the preceding chapter. The investigator should be particularly careful in collecting such evidence if the case is a homicide.

A preliminary examination of the gun may indicate how many shots were fired. This information, together with the number of entrance wounds on the body, may reveal the need for a search of spent bullets, including the ones that pass through the body. If any loose bullets are found, they should be collected. If they are embedded in the walls, ceiling or furniture, they should be extracted and retained.

The type of bullets and their markings may help identify the gun. From some weapons spent cartridges are automatically ejected. These as well as shotgun shells should be carefully searched for at the scene. In the absence of a gun at the scene, these cartridges and shells with their identifying information may indicate the type of gun used and may lead to the identification of the particular gun that inflicted the wounds.

Documentation of Findings

In any medicolegal work, documentation of the facts is vitally important. Therefore, from the time the first call is received, records on the case should be maintained. First of all, the date and the time of the call and the name of the party calling should be noted. The name of the decedent, if known, and the address and telephone number of the place where the body is found should be asked for and noted. Careful notes should be made of the details of the circumstances of death and of the observations made at the scene. The general appearance of the location of death should be described. If the gun is present at the scene, its position in relation to the body should be noted as well as its serial number, make, model, caliber, type of action and a description of the ammunition.

ROLE OF THE MEDICAL INVESTIGATOR

When called upon to investigate a death, the role of a medical investigator is to:

1. Pronounce the person dead.
2. Help identify the decedent if his identity is not known.
3. Determine the cause of death.
4. Assist in determining the manner of death (i.e., whether accidental, suicidal, or homicidal).
5. Help establish approximate time of death.
6. In a homicide, assist in identifying the person responsible for death.

In preparation for the investigation, it is advisable to carry a kit with the following articles:
1. Notebook and pen
2. Camera with films and flash
3. Syringe with 4-inch, size 15 needle and containers
4. Thermometer with temperature range of 0° to 120°F
5. Measuring tape
6. Pair of gloves
7. Small plastic bags and labels
8. Flashlight
9. Stethoscope

On arrival at the scene, the medical investigator must identify himself to the person present in charge of the remains. If there is suspicion of foul play, he must call the police, if they are not already there, and work in cooperation with them. He can then proceed with the investigation systematically along the following lines:
1. Obtain information about the circumstances of death and the background of the decedent.
2. Make observations about the overall scene (e.g., room surroundings, clothes, etc.).
3. Photograph the scene and the body before anything is moved, and, if indicated, after the body is moved.
4. Examine the body carefully

The investigator should spend a few moments carefully observing the entire scene without unnecessarily disturbing it while the police work on other aspects of the case such as the search for fingerprints. He should not handle the weapon carelessly lest he erase the assailant's fingerprints and put his own on it. If the case is a homicide and the determination of time of death seems important, rectal temperature of the decedent should be obtained and observations made about weather conditions at the site the body was found. All the facts and findings at the scene should be recorded on a form such as that on page 58.

At the scene of death, one of the first functions of a medical investigator or a coroner is to make sure that the injured person is in fact dead. If the dead person has not been identified, the medical examiner will be able to assist. He will be able to look for identifying features such as tattoos, scars, etc. on the body and will be able to pull out

RECORD OF FACTS AND FINDINGS AT
THE SCENE OF DEATH

Date and Time of Call: Called by:
Name of Decedent: Age: Race: Sex:
Place of Death (Address):
Date and Time of Scene Investigation:
Type of Death (e.g., homicide, accident, etc.):
Body Identified by:

Circumstances of Death: 1. Past Medical History:
                          2. Events Leading to Death:
                          3. Time and Date Decedent Last Seen
                             Alive:
                          4. Time and Date Body Found:
Description of Body: 1. Approximate Height and Weight:
                          2. Clothing:
                          3. Injuries—fatal and nonfatal:
                          4. Livor:
                          5. Rigor:
                          6. Body Temperature
                             (Rectal Temperature):
Probable Cause of Death:
Probable Manner of Death:
Rough Sketch of the Scene:

Name of Person Authorized to Move the Body:

wallet, papers or other identifying materials from the pockets of the decedent's clothes, if this has not already been done.

In most cases the cause of death is obvious, but the examination of the scene can be of great assistance in determining the manner of death. In every part of the world, suicide bears a stigma. For this reason and for the reason of insurance claims, an attempt may be made by members of the family to conceal suicide and make it look as if the death were accidental or natural. In such circumstances the information given by the family members should be carefully evaluated and their reactions appropriately interpreted because of the possibility of alterations made at the scene prior to the arrival of the investigators. Similarly, in criminal cases, the criminal may alter the scene to conceal a homicide. If there is the slightest suspicion of foul play, the case should be treated as homicide until proved otherwise.

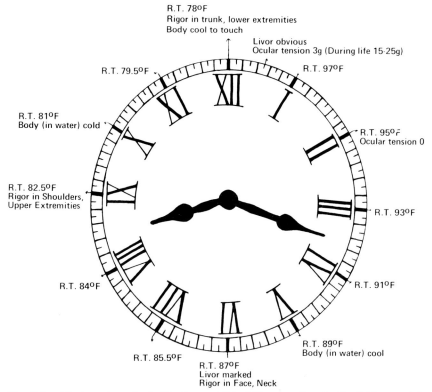

Fig. 5-1. Postmortem clock: Findings at 1 to 12 hours after death; R.T. = rectal temperature.

At the scene of death, a medical investigator is frequently asked at what time death occurred. The determination of the time of death of a homicide victim is often vital, since it may help exclude certain suspects and aid in limiting the investigation to a certain time period. Precise estimation of the time of death is extremely difficult to determine, fiction presentations on television notwithstanding. Because of many variable factors, the estimation of time of death can be made only within broad limits. The best method of approach at the scene is a consideration of the combination of the circumstances of death, the history of the whereabouts of the decedent, the factors affecting the changes in the body after death, and the use of the available methods to determine the time of death. The rate of cooling of the body after death is generally accepted as the most dependable criterion in estimating the lapse of time during the first 12 to 18 hours after death. The reliability of rigor mortis as a criterion for timing of death is influenced by various factors such as metabolic processes of the body and environmental temperature. Ordinarily, the muscles of the face and the neck show rigor about 6 hours after death, the muscles of the shoulders and upper extremities in the next few hours, muscles of the trunk and then the muscles of the lower extremities in about 12 hours. Rigor persists for another 12 hours; then, after about 24 hours, it begins to disappear, disappearing in about 12 hours in the same order it appeared. Some of the changes that can help determine the time of death during the important period of the first 12 hours after death are summarized in a "postmortem clock" (Fig. 5–1).[1]

Collection of Evidence

While the examination of the scene and the body is being made, attention should be paid to the collection of objects of evidential value as described earlier. The police and the medical investigator should work together in this task. Patient search can be rewarding.

The body of a 58-year-old white male was left in the Intracoastal Waterway a few feet from the bank. It appeared that the body had been dragged after it was unloaded at the scene. From the bank out towards the road there was a trail of blood and brain tissues over a distance of 62 feet in rocks and sand. The man had been shot and beaten on the head and the brain tissue had extruded through multiple fractures of the skull. Careful examination of the spots of blood and brain tissue along the entire trail revealed a bullet in one of the fragments of brain.

STATEMENTS AT THE SCENE

Occasionally, the scene of death is surrounded by curious observers and representatives from the news media. With the help of police, the area can be roped off so that unhindered investigation can be carried out. Always refrain from answering questions from the casual observer and exercise great caution in answering questions from the press. It is permissible to state the cause and manner of death if there is no doubt about them. However, if the circumstances are not clear, it is unwise to speculate publicly or to discuss theories about the motive of the criminal in a case of homicide. It is best to say that the investigation is not completed and that no conclusions have been reached. As far as the relationship with the law enforcement agents involved in the investigation is concerned, the medical investigator should cooperate fully, and freely exchange information.

REFERENCE

1. Fatteh, A.: Handbook of Forensic Pathology. Philadelphia, J. B. Lippincott, 1973.

6

Photography in the Investigation of Firearm Crime

In olden days, documentation of crime was done with descriptions, diagrams, maps and models. In modern times, photography has formed an important dimension in investigation. The law enforcement agents and other investigators have become increasingly aware of the significance of photographs in various phases of investigation. The judicial courts are allowing the use of photographs, both black-and-white and color, more frequently. Photography is a good form of communication, and it has often played an important role in documenting crimes and in getting convictions.

Photographs provide a true-to-life pictorial view of the scene of the crime, of the wounds on the body and of all articles of evidential value. They not only serve the investigator to refresh his memory but also provide a clear concept of the details of investigation to the judge and the jurors hearing the case. For these reasons, every crime must be documented with photographs. Ordinarily, a general-purpose camera with flash equipment will be sufficient. For most of the large-object photography in medicolegal investigations a 35 mm camera with color negative film is adequate because color and black-and-white prints can be satisfactorily made from such a film. At times, however, photographing of special features or of small objects will require different cameras, lenses and films.

In view of the importance of photographs related to a criminal investigation, the photographs should, as far as possible, be taken by a police officer trained in crime photography and fully equipped for the job. Many police departments have trained photographers on the staff, and these are summoned whenever a crime is suspected or is known to have been committed. The photographer responding to a call to a crime scene should carry all necessary equipment and ample films.

In this chapter, details of the techniques of photography are not discussed. Rather, the emphasis is on the investigational aspects.

PHOTOGRAPHS OF THE SCENE OF SHOOTING

As in all other phases of crime, photographs can be invaluable in documenting the details of the scene of shooting. The investigator photographing the scene of crime should take a series of photographs to document all aspects of the case. The photographs should be taken in such a way that they would contribute to a clear understanding of the crime when finished photographs are examined at a future date The photographs should depict the relative positions of various objects at the scene of crime and they should show the points of reference clearly. In order to cover the details of the scene, photographs from various angles must be taken. A set of photographs must be taken before anything is moved. Photography of the scene after various objects are moved is another important aspect of investigation. In a case of a firearm fatality the gun, cartridge cases, shells or bullets may be found under the victim's body or they may be concealed by pieces of furniture and other objects.

At the scene of a crime, a good principle for the photographer to remember is that he should never rush into taking photographs. A few moments of thinking and planning will yield much better results. The other good principle is to take too many rather than too few photographs.

In a case of criminal shooting, photographs of the following areas are important:

Overall Scene

The general view of the scene of crime will be helpful in explaining the relative locations of various articles of evidence and of the body of the victim. Therefore, several shots from different angles and positions should be taken to cover the entire area of investigation. The photographs should include only the objects of evidential value found at the scene of crime. The articles of equipment carried by the investigators and unnecessary persons should be excluded from the photographs.

The Victim's Body

The location and the posture of the victim at the scene of crime can best be documented with photographs. The main objective of such photographs is to show the body in the posture and condition found and also to show its location in relation to the items of evidence such as the gun, bullets, cartridge cases, etc. (Fig. 6-1). It is not necessary to obtain close-up photographs of gunshot wounds or bullet holes in the clothing because this can be better done later in the autopsy room.

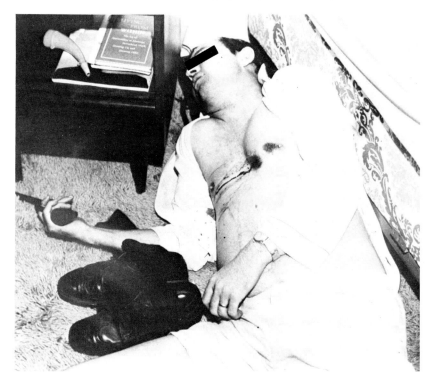

Fig. 6-1. A scene photograph showing important details.

The Articles of Evidence

After photographing the general scene and the victim's body, attention should be directed to photographing the articles of evidence. At the scene of a shooting there may be the weapon, spent and unspent ammunition, portions of the victim's and assailant's clothing, hair, blood, broken glass and broken furniture. These should be photographed before and after they are moved.

Locations of Evidential Value

In addition to movable objects, there may be points of evidential significance at the scene of a shooting. For instance, there may be bullet holes in the walls, floor, ceiling or in the furniture. The victim's or the assailant's foot or shoe impressions may be present. There may also be trails of blood or tissue giving some clue to the movements of the victim or the assailant.

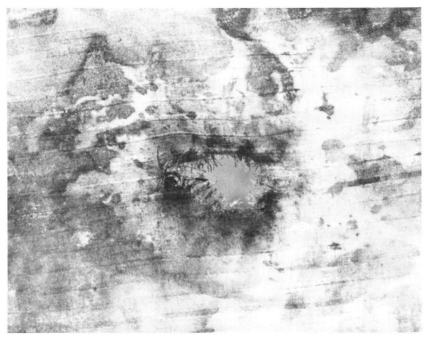

Fig. 6-2.   Clothing showing a bullet hole with gunpowder.

Photographs of Fingerprints

Fingerprints often play an important role in an investigation. Every effort should be made to photograph fingerprints at the scene of crime. Of course, a professional photographer versed in the technique of photographing fingerprints using a special camera should be assigned this task.

PHOTOGRAPHY IN THE AUTOPSY ROOM

In many jurisdictions the role of the investigating police officer comes to an end when the body of the victim of a criminal assault is moved to the autopsy room. Such a tradition is undesirable. The police officer who investigates the scene of crime should attend the autopsy on the body of the victim. This will give him an opportunity to collect articles of evidence from the doctor and also to take photographs. Together the pathologist and the law enforcement agent should take the following photographs:

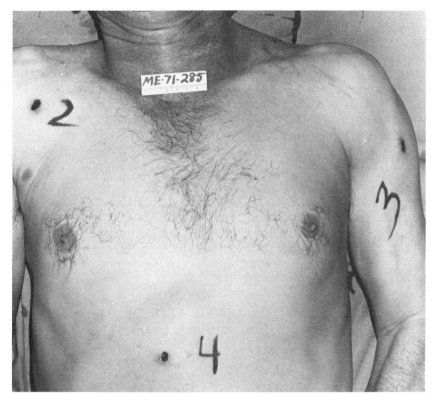

Fig. 6-3. A photograph showing multiple gunshot wounds.

Photographs of the Body in the Condition Received

Before undressing or cleaning the body and before the autopsy is commenced, the body should be photographed to document the condition of the body when received.

Identification Photographs

Sometimes the identification of the body is challenged in the court of law if such an identification is based on body tags. In order to avoid such challenges, it is suggested that the pathologist make a photograph of the decedent's full face (after it is cleaned) with an identifying label. A profile photograph of the decedent's face may also be taken. Such photographs will enable the pathologist to say that he performed the autopsy on the decedent shown in the photograph. An additional

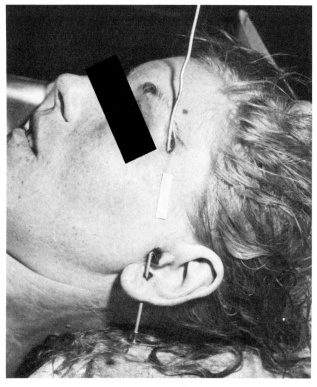

Fig. 6-4.   Entrance, exit, re-entrance and re-exit wounds lined up with a probe.

photograph showing the decedent's face with the prosector standing nearby is taken in some jurisdictions.

Photographs of the Clothes

After the body is unclothed, important areas of the clothing should be photographed. In particular, entrance and exit bullet holes should be photographed with identifying labels. The bullet holes in the clothing may be photographed with corresponding gunshot wounds in the skin. For further clarity, individual bullet holes in the clothing may be identified with numbers assigned to corresponding gunshot wounds on the body (Fig. 6-2).

Photographs of the External Gunshot Wounds

After the areas of the wounds are cleaned, photographs of all entrance and exit gunshot wounds should be taken with identifying labels and rulers. First an overall shot should be taken to show as many wounds as possible and then close-up photographs of individual wounds should be taken. To match these with the descriptions of the wounds, it is advisable to assign a number to each wound. Such a number, identification label and the ruler should be included in the photograph (Fig. 6-3). There should be no hesitation to shave the area if the wound is concealed by hair. If it is possible to document photographically the direction of fire, a probe may be inserted in the wound and photographed. The probe extending from the entrance wound to the exit wound will depict the direction of fire well (Fig. 6-4). Many photographers neglect to place the labels and rulers in a uniform way. They place the labels in different directions—horizontally, vertically, obliquely and even upside down in relation to the wound. This invariably makes it difficult to identify from close-up photographs as to which is the upper, lower, right or left margin of the wound. If the label is always placed above or below the wound and always perpendicular to the long axis of the body, no matter what area of the body is photographed, the orientation of the photograph is rendered easy. Photographs taken with such uniformity are easy to present and easy to explain while testifying in court.

All injuries other than the gunshot wounds should also be photographically recorded even if they are minor in nature. Every area photographed should include an identifying label, and whenever indicated, a ruler should be included.

In addition to the photographs of the injuries, identifying features such as tattoos and scars and other significant features on the exterior of the body should also be photographed.

Photographs of Internal Injuries

Photographs of the internal organs will help demonstrate the extent of injuries and locations of the bullets. With a pointer or other marker included they will also serve to indicate the direction of fire.

Photographs of Evidence Removed from the Body

The internal examination of the body may yield bullets, pellets and wadding. These may be photographed in the autopsy room or later in the laboratory (Fig. 6-5). At times fibers of clothing may be found in the track of the wound.

Photomicrographs of Skin Wounds

Portions of skin with gunshot wounds may be removed for making histological sections. The microscopic sections of skin may give information about the range of fire and also indicate whether the wound is

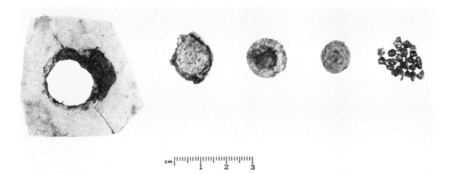

Fig. 6-5. A photograph showing pellets, wads and fabric removed from the head, and a portion of the skull with a bullet hole.

an entrance wound or an exit wound. Various details of the changes in the wounds are discussed in Chapter 8. The pathologist may desire to illustrate with photographs such changes in court to substantiate his verbal testimony.

Photographs of X-rays

The use of x-rays in the investigation of firearm fatalities is becoming increasingly common. Details of the role of x-rays are discussed elsewhere in this book. Whenever x-rays are made in the autopsy room these may be photographed for convenience of presentation of evidence in court.

SPECIAL PHOTOGRAPHIC TECHNIQUES

In the investigation of a crime, especially one involving shooting, the following special techniques can be used.

Process Film

Process film can be used to outline the powder residue on clothing. This film with its great contrast effect can yield satisfactory identification and demarcation of gunpowder residue on light clothing.

Infrared Photographs

This technique is particularly useful when one has to deal with identification of powder residue around a bullet hole in dark clothing. The infrared film gives good contrast, and it is easy to visualize gunpowder residue particles in dark clothing when naked-eye examination of the clothing fails to reveal anything. Technical details are discussed in an Eastman Kodak Company publication.[1]

Soft X-Rays

The presence of lead fouling and particles of metals in clothing can be detected and x-rayed with a soft x-ray apparatus. Radiographs made with soft x-rays of areas showing bullet holes in clothing will reveal the metallic fouling. Stone and Petty have recently (1974) used soft x-ray radiography technique to detect gunshot residues and to distinguish entrance bullet holes from exit bullet holes in clothing.[6] This technique can also be used to study the entrance and exit gunshot wounds in the skin after it is removed from the body.

Comparison Camera

Comparison microscopes are frequently used to make comparisons of bullets recovered from the scene of crime or from the victim's body with the test-fired bullets. They are also used to study various markings such as firing pin impressions, breechlock marks, magazine marks, extractor marks and ejector marks on cartridges. Some of these microscopes have camera attachment so that photomicrographs can be made of the objects under study (see Fig. 3-4). The camera is mounted in such a way that the images in the microscope can be viewed by eyes without removing the camera. Once the field of interest is found under the microscope, the camera can be swung in and the objects photographed. Although comparison cameras are the best means to photograph details on the bullets and cartridges, such photographs are not commonly used in courts because verbal or written reports are easily accepted in courts and because such photographs are not easily understood by juries.

Scanning Electron Microscope Photography

The scanning electron microscope (SEM) has been used in recent years for examining firing pin impressions[2,3] and for microstriation characterization of bullets.[4] The examination of copper-jacketed bullets using SEM by the latter group of workers has led them to conclude that consistent sets of microstriations are present within each striation on a bullet and that these microstriations are a potential means for comparison of evidence bullets and test fired bullets. The SEM photomicrographs of the microstriations are thus useful aids in the investigation of a shooting crime.

MOVIE FILMS

Relevant movie pictures are rarely available for use in the solution of a crime or for presentation in court. The only time useful movies may be made incidentally is when a national figure is shot. The assassinations by gunfire of President J. F. Kennedy, Lee Harvey Oswald and Senator

R. F. Kennedy were filmed and some of the films proved to be invaluable.

In an important case, if movie films are made to document the findings of an investigation with a view to use them in court all relevant information about the type of film, speed of exposure and the date and time of filming should be noted.[5]

USE OF PHOTOGRAPHS AS TEACHING AIDS

The most common use of crime photographs is for teaching. Color slides are useful for teaching law enforcement agents, pathologists, coroners, medical examiners and attorneys.

USE OF PHOTOGRAPHS IN COURT

Of the many photographs the investigators take, only a few will be required to be presented in court. The police investigator or the pathologist should pick out only those photographs that are going to make a meaningful contribution in the court. All photographs that are immaterial or irrelevant should be excluded. The photographs to be presented in the court, especially at a jury trial, should not be inflammatory, for they might incite prejudice or sympathy. They should be free from distortion and should not misrepresent the facts. Any photographs showing artefacts or giving misleading information should not be submitted as exhibits.

It had been customary until recently to use black-and-white photographs in court. Color photographs showing blood were vehemently objected to by many defending attorneys and rejected by judges on the ground that they were inflammatory. However, in recent years more and more courts are allowing the use of color photographs to illustrate the testimony.

Photographs serve various useful purposes in court:

1. The witness will be able to refresh his memory of his findings by looking at the photographs while in the witness box.

2. The pathologist will be able to establish the identity of the decedent on whom he performed the autopsy by presenting the photographs of the decedent's face.

3. The witness will be able to explain his findings to the jurors conveniently, and in turn the jurors will be able to understand the testimony better if it is illustrated with photographs.

4. The photographs provide true-to-life picture of the investigative findings to the jurors and they enhance the credibility of the verbal testimony of the witnesses.

REFERENCES

1. Eastman Kodak Company: Applied Infrared Photography. Publication No. M-28 CAT 101 8365. Rochester, New York, 1972.
2. Grove, C. A., Judd, G. and Horn, R.: Examination of firing pin impressions by scanning electron microscopy. J. For. Sci., *17*:659, 1972.
3. ————: Evaluation of SEM potential in the examination of shotgun and rifle firing pin impressions. J. For. Sci., *19*:441, 1974.
4. Judd, G., Sabo, J., Hamilton, W., Ferriss, S. and Horn, R.: SEM microstriation characterization of bullets and contaminant particle identification. J. For. Sci., *19*:798, 1974.
5. Prescott, P. S.: The Role of Photography in Crime Investigation. *In* Keith Simpson (ed.): Modern Trends in Forensic Medicine. New York, Appleton-Century-Crofts, 1967.
6. Stone, I. C. and Petty, C. S.: Examination of gunshot residues. J. For. Sci., *19*:784, 1974.

7

The Role of X-Rays in the Investigation

X-radiation was discovered by Wilhelm Conrad Roentgen in 1895, in the city of Wurzburg. Within only three months after Roentgen's announcement of the discovery, the first x-ray department was started in Glasgow. In recent years x-ray methods have found applications in many fields, and the use of x-rays in forensic investigations is by no means uncommon in the United States. In most other countries, however, radiology is not used as a routine tool in the investigation of medicolegal cases. In some countries it is rare to find a mortuary equipped with an x-ray apparatus, and hence radiology is used only in special cases.

GENERAL USES OF X-RAYS IN MEDICOLEGAL CASES

Radiological examinations can be of immense help in the investigation of a variety of medicolegal cases. X-rays can give clues to the identity of an individual by determining the age, the height and the sex of the person or by detecting old fractures, infective changes or congenital bony changes. Mann and Fatteh (1968) have described a case in which the identity of a murder victim, in an advanced state of decomposition, was made for legal purposes by postmortem x-rays.[4] The x-rays showed a fracture of the zygomatic arch caused during life by a bullet (Fig. 7-1). Antemortem x-rays were available for comparison. X-rays may also aid in identification of a person by demonstrating fingerprints.

X-rays are useful, also, in the investigation of the cases of battered child syndrome, burns, drowning and decomposition. For instance, in one case, x-rays of a markedly decomposed body of a man led to the detection of a BB shot in the orbital region (Fig. 7-2). The history of an accidental shooting and lodgement of the shot in the eye, together with other clues, led to positive identification of the deceased.

Radiology may provide useful information in the cases of air embolism, pneumothorax and hemothorax. These and other general uses of radiology in forensic pathology have been described by Fatteh and Mann.[1]

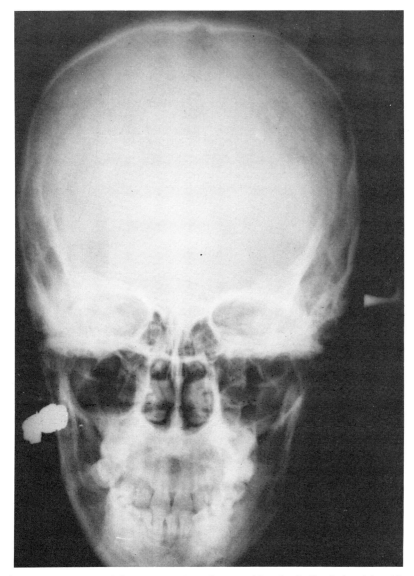

Fig. 7-1. Fracture of the zygomatic arch caused by the bullet led to identification of decomposed remains.

USES OF X-RAYS IN SHOOTING CASES

Use of X-Ray Examination at the Scene of Shooting

X-rays can be of value in various ways in the investigation of firearm injuries and fatalities. The investigation of a firearm injury or fatality begins at the scene of the shooting. In most instances, there is no need

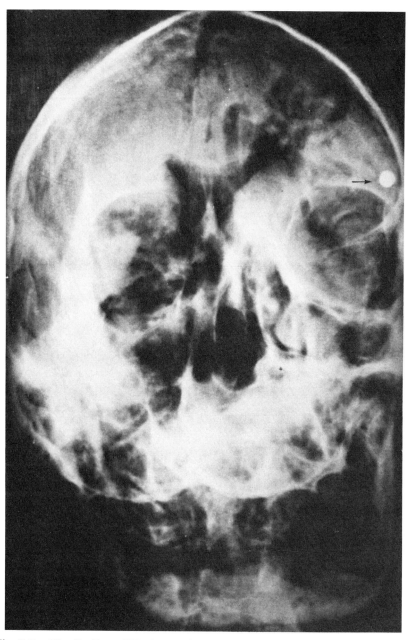

Fig. 7-2. The finding of BB shot in the eye during a routine x-ray examination led to identification of the deceased.

to make x-rays at the scene of the shooting. In some cases, however, the availability of a portable x-ray machine can greatly assist in localizing the fired missiles in the body and in other objects such as mattresses,

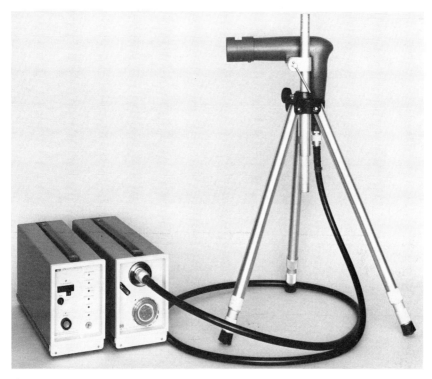

Fig. 7-3.   Portable x-ray system: Hewlett-Packard Model 43501A (Courtesy of Hewlett-Packard Company).

furniture, wooden floor, etc. Such a localization of missiles will help in determining the number of shots fired and it will assist in retrieving the missiles embedded in the objects at the scene of the shooting. A crime laboratory or a medical examiner's office handling a large number of cases should be equipped with a portable x-ray machine. Several small lightweight units are available in the market. Two such machines are shown in Figures 7-3 and 7-4. In the absence of permanent equipment in the autopsy room, such a machine will serve a useful purpose.

X-Ray Examinations in the Autopsy Room

It is advisable to x-ray the body of the victim of gunshot wounds prior to autopsy if facilities are available. X-rays will readily give information about the location of the missiles in the body, number of missiles in the body, angle and direction of fire, depth of the wounds and the type of firearm (i.e., rifled weapon or shotgun).

Localization of the Missile.   One of the most important uses of x-rays is localization of the missile in the body. Recovery of the bullet

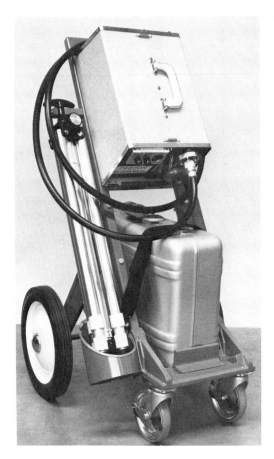

Fig. 7-4. Portable x-ray machine: Hewlett-Packard Model 43802 (Courtesy of Hewlet-Packard Company).

can be very difficult and time-consuming without x-rays. Lodgement of the bullet in the face, neck, pelvis or spine can make retrieval of the missile especially difficult. X-ray localization of the bullet will greatly aid in removing the bullet lodged in such an area. Anterior and lateral films of the general area in which the bullet is suspected to be lodged save a considerable amount of the pathologist's time and effort in the search of the missile. Sometimes it is necessary to make several films to localize the bullet.

Occasionally, radiological examination does not reveal the presence of a missile in the general direction of fire in the body. Deflection of the missile after it hits a bone in the body may make its retrieval at autopsy difficult without x-rays. Also, a missile may gain access to the blood stream and be carried away as an embolus. In such circumstances, the finding of the missile without x-rays may be extremely difficult if not impossible.

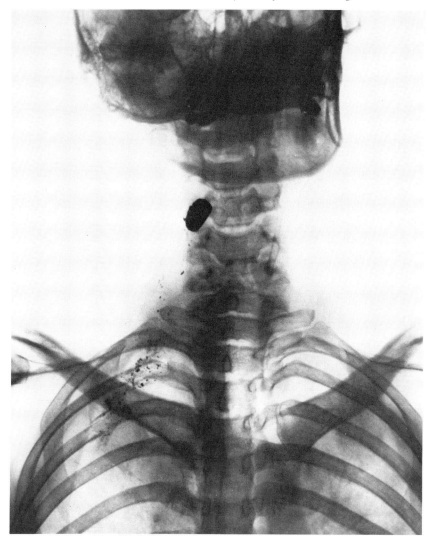

Fig. 7-5. An x-ray showing direction of fire (Courtesy of Hewlett-Packard Company).

Number of Bullets in the Body. With proper x-rays, the number of bullets in the body will be immediately known. In a case with no exit wounds, the number of bullets in the body should correspond with the number of entrance wounds. The absence of a missile in the body as revealed by x-rays in a case with an entrance wound will prompt the examiner to look for an exit wound. Sometimes x-rays reveal unexpected information. In one case of a firearm victim with a single en-

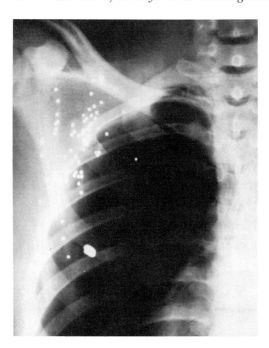

Fig. 7-6. An x-ray showing shotgun pellets as well as a small caliber missile (Courtesy of H. L. Taylor, M.D.).

trance gunshot wound and no exit wound, radiology revealed the presence of two bullets in the body. The shooting had occurred at a "party" where at least three and probably five different firearms were involved. It was important in this case to recover both bullets and determine their role in the cause of death. Without x-rays, one of the bullets might have perhaps been missed. In another instance, two bullets were fired into the victim's body through one point by an assailant. Routine x-rays helped retrieve both of the bullets. A tandem bullet may cause one entrance wound whereas there may be two bullets within the body. Without x-rays one of them may be missed.

Angle and Direction of Fire.   Very often x-rays provide information that can help determine the angle and direction of fire. The localization of metallic particles at or near the point of entry and the point of lodgement of the bullet will give an idea about the angle and direction of fire (Fig. 7-5).

Depth of Wound.   The depth of a particular wound caused by a bullet can be evaluated from its course and the point of its final lodgement in the body.

Type of Firearm.   X-rays will, by detecting bullets or pellets in the body, give an immediate clue as to whether the firearm involved was a rifled weapon or a shotgun. If more than one gun was used, x-rays may indicate the type of weapons. For instance, in one case of shooting,

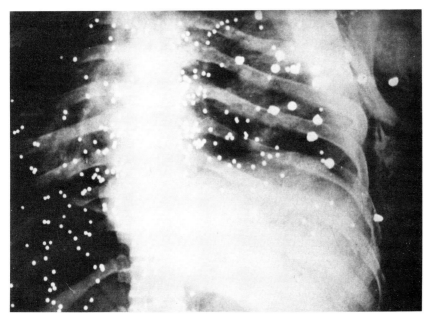

Fig. 7-7. An x-ray showing pellets of two sizes (Courtesy of Page Hudson, M.D.).

x-rays revealed not only shotgun pellets but also a small caliber missile (Fig. 7-6). In another instance, shotgun pellets of different sizes were discovered by radiological examination (Fig. 7-7). A case is described in chapter 13 in which an x-ray of the head of a shooting victim showed a 0.22 caliber missile and tiny pellets from a No. 12 bird shot (See Fig. 13-1).

From the examination of the x-rays, one should not venture an opinion on the caliber of the bullet in the body from its size in the x-rays. The size of the shadow of a bullet will vary with its distance from the film.

X-Rays in the Detection of Secret Homicide

X-Rays of Skeletonized Remains. X-ray examination of skeletonized remains may reveal the presence of missiles or pellets lodged in the bones or loose in the remains. Bullets may cause fractures of bones. In such cases small fragments of metal may be found along the missile track in the bone or at the site of fracture. Retrieval of such fragments of metal and determination of their composition may help identify a missile found with the remains.

X-Rays of Decomposed Bodies. Whenever the circumstances of death are unclear, all decomposing remains should be x-rayed to rule out the possibility of violence, especially shooting. Such practice of routine x-raying brings out frequent surprises to the forensic pathologist. For example, in one instance, initial examination of an adipocered body of a woman dumped at the border of a cemetery raised no hope of answers to medicolegal questions. The x-rays of the remains, however, revealed a shotgun blast of the head. This finding, together with other observations, eventually led to the arrest and conviction of a man for murder.

Routine fluoroscopy of a man who was claimed to have "dropped dead" and whose body tissues were extensively eaten up by hogs presented unexpected findings. The man had been shot three times from three different distances by a shotgun.[5]

X-Rays of Burned Bodies.   One of the most important objectives of an autopsy on a burned body is the exclusion of the possibility of foul play. X-rays of the remains can be invaluable in the investigation as illustrated by the following cases.

A middle-aged, chronic alcoholic was found dead in a dilapidated abode that was often used by chronic alcoholics. His charred body was discovered after the fire, which destroyed the abode, was extinguished. The circumstances pointed to this being an accidental death. However, x-rays of the body, prior to postmortem examination, revealed a bullet in the spine. Dissection for the removal of the bullet showed recent hemorrhages along the track of the missile.

On another occasion, severely burned bodies of a couple—husband and wife—were found in a burned house. Investigation indicated the possibility of murder-suicide. X-rays revealed one bullet in the woman's head and two in the man's. At the autopsy, the bullet in the woman's head was found in the brain and the point of entry of the bullet was in the back of the head. The autopsy on the man revealed such beveling of the skull as to indicate that one bullet had entered the cranium from the right side of the head and the other from the left. This was a double murder.

Use of X-Rays in Fingerprinting

Fingerprints are one of the most important aids in the investigation of firearm deaths. They can help in identifying a criminal and in associating him with a gun used by him in a crime. Visualization and demonstration of fingerprints on various objects and even on human skin may be aided by x-ray techniques. The methodology has been detailed by Graham.[2] He has also discussed the use of grenz rays in the fingerprint investigations.

Use of X-Ray Diffraction

X-rays can also be useful in the identification of bullet holes. Photographic methods using soft x-rays have been applied to detect lead in certain cases. Krishnan and Nichol have described a method of identification of bullet holes by neutron activation analysis (NAA) and autoradiography of metallic deposits around these holes.[3] The method helps to identify antimony and copper deposits at the bullet holes. By this method it is possible to say whether the bullet was copper-jacketed or not. The authors indicate that the method is simple, fast, effective and nondestructive. Neutron activation autoradiography has also been used by these authors to identify bullet holes in clothing and to estimate the distance of fire.

The use of x-rays in the study of wound ballistics should also be mentioned. X-ray photographs of bullets passing through a material, such as gelatin, which simulates human tissue may help to illustrate the destructive effects of the bullets.

IDENTIFICATION OF X-RAYS

Whenever x-rays are made either at the scene of investigation or in the autopsy room, they should bear proper identifying data. The x-ray plate itself should either have the name of the victim or the number assigned to the case with the date of examination. A mark in one corner of the plate indicating right or left side of the body of the victim should also be included. Such information will greatly facilitate testimony in court at a later date.

REFERENCES

1. Fatteh, A. and Mann, G. T.: The role of radiology in forensic pathology. Medicine, Science and Law, 9:24, 1969.
2. Graham, D.: The Use of X-Ray Techniques in Forensic Investigations. London, Churchill Livingstone, 1973.
3. Krishnan, S. S. and Nichol, R. C.: Identification of bullet holes by neutron activation analysis and autoradiography. J. For. Sci., 13:519, 1968.
4. Mann, G. T. and Fatteh, A.: The role of radiology in the identification of human remains. J. For. Sci. Soc., 8:67, 1968.
5. Morgan, T. A. and Harris, M. C.: The use of x-rays as an aid to medicolegal investigation. J. For. Med., 1:28, 1954.

8

Entrance Gunshot Wounds

BASIC QUESTIONS

In the investigation of a firearm injury or fatality, the study of the entrance gunshot wounds can provide answers to several important questions. Although it is easy to interpret entrance wounds in most of the cases, in some instances the interpretation is far from easy. No amount of reading will make one an expert in the interpretation of gunshot wounds. The literature can only provide guidelines. Practical experience is mandatory for gaining the expertise essential in the interpretation of gunshot wounds.

The examination of gunshot wounds should be aimed at answering the following questions in the cases of a fatal shooting:
1. Is a wound being examined a gunshot wound?
2. Is the wound an entrance wound or an exit wound?
3. What type of gun caused the wound?
4. What was the range of fire?
5. What was the direction of fire?
6. What were the relative positions of the gun and the victim?
7. Did the gunshot wound cause death?
8. How many times was the decedent shot?

Considerations of various aspects of firearm injuries by the pathologist will enable him to answer these questions.

Is the Wound Being Examined a Gunshot Wound?

This basic question might at first appear superfluous. However, at times the features of a wound are such that it is simply not possible to identify it as a gunshot wound by mere external examination of the wound itself. A stab wound caused by a round pointed instrument may resemble a gunshot wound. A bullet that passes through glass or some other object and then strikes the body may create a wound that may resemble a laceration (Fig. 8-1). A bullet that ricochets after striking

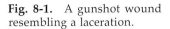

Fig. 8-1. A gunshot wound resembling a laceration.

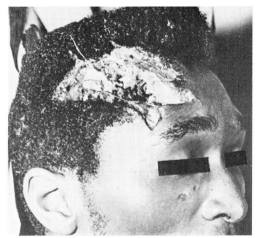

another object and then enters the body may cause a wound with no characteristics of a typical entrance gunshot wound. Tumbling bullets may cause wounds that may be difficult to recognize as bullet wounds.

In situations when helpful criteria are not present, additional considerations such as the circumstances of death, study of x-rays and the findings of internal examination will have to be taken into account. The history of the shooting, the finding of a bullet or bullet fragments in the x-rays and the nature of the internal injuries together with the recovery of the bullet or its fragments will aid in establishing that the external injury is a gunshot wound.

Is the Wound an Entrance Wound or an Exit Wound?

The discussion in this chapter and in the next deals with general appearances of entrance and exit gunshot wounds, respectively. This general information will guide the examiner in drawing his conclusions. However, despite all care in the examination, there will still be instances in which correct interpretation of a wound will be difficult, if not impossible. The cases that create confusion are the ones with multiple entrance and exit wounds. A particularly perplexing situation may be created if multiple bullets have entered, exited, re-entered and re-exited. In difficult cases, in addition to studying the gross features and reconstructing the pathways of the bullets, it may be necessary to make additional studies. These may include tests for detection of nitrites and nitrates, and microscopic examination of the sections of wounds. It is most advisable to analyze the case carefully and completely before the body is released.

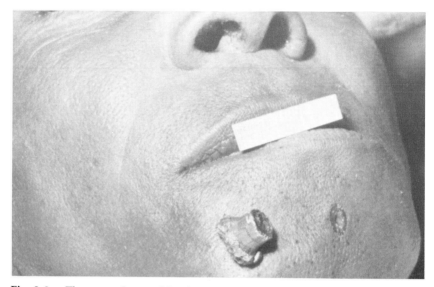

Fig. 8-2. The wound caused by the 0.38 caliber bullet is much smaller than the bullet itself.

What Type of Gun Caused the Wound?

The nature of a wound generally indicates the type of gun that inflicted it. The wounds caused by shotguns are usually easy to identify. As for the wounds caused by rifled weapons, the size of the wound is not always helpful in determining the caliber or type of weapon (pistol, revolver, rifle). In fact, the size of the wound can be misleading (Fig. 8-2). The diameter of the wound may be smaller, greater or equal to the diameter of the bullet. Therefore, one must give a guarded opinion about the caliber of the bullet from the examination of the wound (Fig. 8-3).

What Was the Range of Fire?

The answer to this question is frequently important in homicidal shootings. Also, occasionally, it is important to exclude the possibility of suicide. The appearances of wounds caused from various distances are discussed elsewhere in this chapter.

What Was the Direction of Fire?

The direction of fire may be determined from the external examination of the entrance wound and from the direction of the bullet track within the body. A round bullet hole will indicate perpendicular hit

Fig. 8-3. The entrance wound caused by the 0.32 caliber bullet is much smaller than the bullet itself.

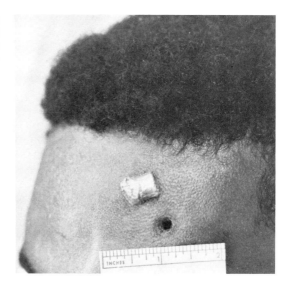

and an abrasion extending from the margin of a wound will indicate that the shot was fired at an angle from the side of the abrasion (see below). However, a tumbling bullet may hit the body along its side and may create an oval or an oblong wound with greater abrading of one of the margins of the wound. A line between the point of entry of the bullet and the point of exit or the site of lodgement of the bullet will indicate the direction of fire. Confusion may, however, be created if the bullet is deflected after it strikes a bone.

What Were the Relative Positions of the Gun and the Victim?

From the examination of the wounds the pathologist may, in some instances, be able to reconstruct the relative positions of the firearm and the victim. Not only that, but sometimes it is also possible to draw conclusions about the posture of the victim at the time he was shot. In the following instance, the location of an entrance gunshot wound on the body and the site of lodgement of the bullet in the body vividly explained the posture of the victim at the time of shooting.

A 20-year-old male was shot with a 0.38 caliber revolver by a girl. An entrance gunshot wound was found on the outer aspect of the lower third on the left arm (Fig. 8-4). No exit wound was present. X-rays of the body revealed the bullet in the chest. The track of the bullet extended from the point of entry in the arm towards the shoulder and continued through the axillary tissues to the third left rib in the mid-axillary line. The bullet entered the chest after fracturing that rib. This pathway of the bullet clearly implied a raised position of the victim's arm

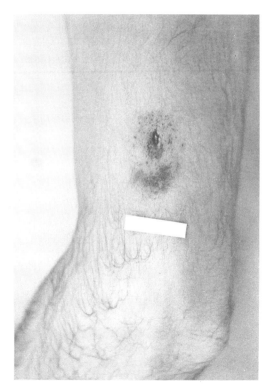

Fig. 8-4. A gunshot wound showing abrasion in its lower margin.

at the time of the shooting. The nature of the abrasion in the lower margin of the entrance gunshot wound also supported such a position of the arm.

Did the Gunshot Wound Cause Death?

This question may be posed under three circumstances: first, when it is suspected that an injury that looks like a gunshot wound may have been caused by an object other than a bullet; secondly, when a victim has sustained multiple gunshot wounds from bullets fired by different guns; and thirdly, when a victim dies a long time after the shooting. In the first instance, the correct interpretation of the wound answers the question. Several pointed objects can cause injuries that may resemble entrance gunshot wounds. The examination of the external wound, its track within the body and the presence or absence of a missile within the body will settle the issue. In the second instance, it would be important to determine which missile was responsible for the fatal injuries. The identification of the pathways of the bullets and the recovery of the missiles will assist in the final disposition of the case. Finally, when the death is delayed after an incident of a shooting, the pathologist will

Fig. 8-5. A contact wound caused by a 0.22 caliber Saturday Night Special showing flame effect.

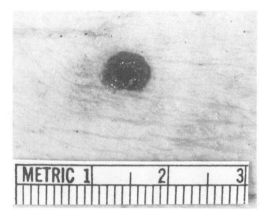

have to establish whether the death was from the complications of the firearm injuries or from unrelated conditions.

How Many Times Was the Decedent Shot?

When multiple shots are fired, one or more bullets may hit the victim. In such situations correct identification of entrance gunshot wounds should be made to determine the number of times the victim was shot. A single bullet may enter and exit more than once, causing multiple wounds. Unless the entrance and the re-entrance wounds are identified and all wounds are correctly lined up, a wrong conclusion about the number of shots fired may be drawn.

ENTRANCE GUNSHOT WOUNDS: CAUSE AND EFFECT

In order to understand the logistics of various appearances of entrance gunshot wounds, it is important for the investigator to be versed in the mechanics of gunfire and the components of the fired shot.

Various events take place in rapid succession as the trigger of a loaded gun is pulled. The primer is first detonated by heat created by the strike of the firing pin. This sets off the powder charge in the cartridge. When the cartridge explodes, the components of the gunfire that cause informative changes on the skin or the clothing are *hot gases, smoke, flame, gunpowder, metallic fragments* and the *bullet* or *pellets*. In addition, *wadding* in shotgun shells will also cause injuries. If the gun is held in contact with the skin, *muzzle* impressions may be caused by impact or pressure. The effects caused by these components are discussed here.

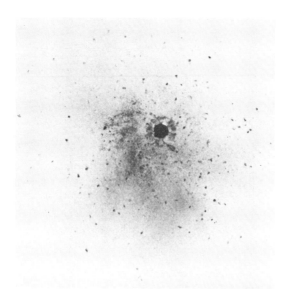

Fig. 8-6. A gunshot
wound showing powder
stippling and smoke
smudging.

Flame Effect: Burning

Burning of the gunpowder produces a flame at the muzzle. The flame
extends to a certain distance. It usually does not extend beyond a distance of about 6 inches with most of the guns used in crime. With a
pistol or revolver, the flame is often less than 3 inches long. Therefore, if
the victim is shot from a distance of less than 6 inches, flame effect may
be seen on the target. The flame causes a burn of the skin in the form of
scorching or charring (Fig. 8-5). If the target area bears hair, this is
singed by the flame. Within the range of the flame, smoke smudging
and gunpowder tattooing will also be seen. In contact wounds, the
flame causes burning of the margins of the wound. Burning of the
tissue causes drying and stiffening of the margins of the wound.

Smoke Effect: Smudging

When a gun is fired, combustion of the gunpowder used produces
gases. The black powder, for instance, produces carbon dioxide (50%),
nitrogen (35%), carbon monoxide (10%), hydrogen sulphide (3%), hydrogen (2%) and traces of methane and oxygen.[2] Smokeless powder
produces much less smoke than black gunpowder. Smoke is light, and
after it leaves the muzzle it does not travel as far as the gunpowder does
and cannot penetrate the target. Therefore, the smoke effect is seen
mainly on the surface of the target. When the smoke effect is present on
the skin, it is in the form of blackening as seen in scorching of the skin;
this is called smoke *smudging*. Smoke forms a blackish-gray film on the

surface of the skin. This can be removed by rubbing or washing. The degree of smoke effect varies with the gun, ammunition and the range of fire. Smoke smudging may be seen with distances of up to 12 inches (Fig. 8-6).

Gunpowder Effect: Tattooing or Stippling

Gunpowder, when ignited, produces a large volume of hot gases within the chamber of the gun. High pressure caused by these gases propels the projectile out of the gun. The propellant commonly used is smokeless powder. This usually is in the form of small squares or discs coated with graphite. The powder residue resulting from explosion of smokeless powder is composed of partially burned or unburned powder granules with nitrites and cellulose nitrates mixed with carbonized matter or graphite. If black gunpowder is used as the propellant, the powder residues that can be detected chemically on the target will be nitrites, thiocyanates, thiosulphates, potassium carbonate, potassium sulphate and potassium sulphide.

The pattern of gunpowder entering the target or getting deposited on the target depends to some extent on the type of firearm and ammunition. The distance of fire, however, makes a major difference. If the muzzle is held close to the target, gunpowder particles will enter the tissue. These particles will cause hemorrhage in deeper tissues. In the margins of the wound caused by the entry of the projectile, these particles will form aggregates of hemorrhages. Thus, the margins of the wound will be contused. As the distance of fire increases the area of scatter of gunpowder also increases. Particles of unburned or partially burned particles, being heavier than smoke, travel farther and hence leave features of evidential value at greater distances. Some of the gunpowder particles enter deeper tissues, some get deposited within the dermis, and some get lodged in the epidermis. The particles embedded in the epidermis and the dermis are visible on external examination. The pattern produced by the lodgement of these partially burned or unburned gunpowder particles in the skin is called *tattooing* or *stippling*.

The particles embedded in the dermis, externally visible, cannot be removed by wiping or washing of the skin. Those sticking to the epidermis or lodging in the epidermis superficially can, however, be removed with pressure wiping. When such particles are removed, punctate wounds caused by them can be seen in the skin surface.

Generally speaking, with the firearms commonly used in crime, tattooing or stippling by unburned or partially burned gunpowder particles is seen around the entrance wound if the gun is fired from a distance of less than 24 inches (Fig. 8-7). There is, however, considerable variability from gun to gun. This is clearly seen in the series of photo-

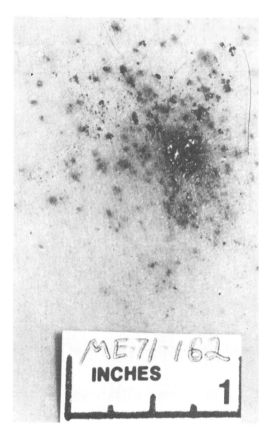

Fig. 8-7. Tattooing by gunpowder particles.

graphs of wounds caused by a 0.357 Smith and Wesson 2½-inch barrel Model 19 and a 0.22 caliber Saturday Night Special from various distances (Figs. 8-8, 8-9, 8-10, 8-11). (These wounds were inflicted on human skin removed from amputated limbs.) If there is a pattern of gunpowder tattooing on the victim's body, test fires with the gun used in the crime and identical ammunition should be made to obtain a similar pattern.

What Is Meant by "Powder Burns"?   The components of a shot that cause blackening of the entrance wound margins are smoke, flame and gunpowder. The smoke smudging causes surface blackening of the skin, the gunpowder causes tattooing, and the flame causes burning of the wound margins. Although all three components do not cause burns, and even though all three components do not contain gunpowder, there is a general tendency to describe the combined effects of smoke, flame and gunpowder as "powder burns." Unless it is clearly understood by all as to what is meant by powder burns there will be misinterpretation

Fig. 8-8. A gunshot wound caused by 0.357 Smith and Wesson Model 19 revolver from a distance of 3 inches.

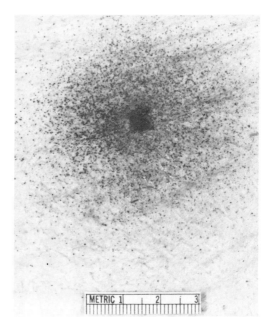

of the phrase "powder burns." Many investigators, for instance, do not consider gunpowder stippling as powder burns. Therefore, while describing the features of entrance wounds the pathologist should be

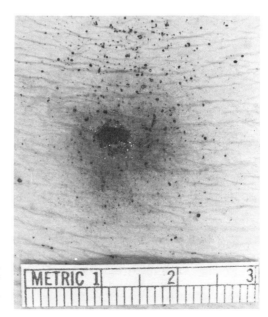

Fig. 8-9. A gunshot wound caused by a 0.22 caliber Saturday Night Special from a distance of 3 inches.

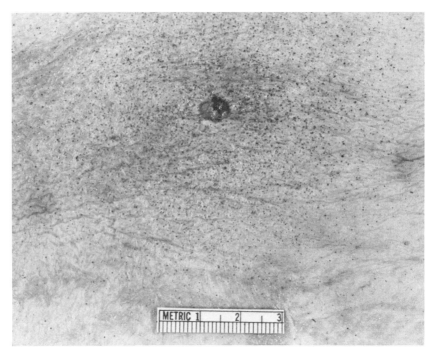

Fig. 8-10.   A gunshot wound caused by a 0.357 Smith and Wesson Model 19 revolver from a distance of 6 inches.

more specific and describe smoke smudging, flame burning and gunpowder tattooing separately so that his reports may not be misunderstood.

Bullet Effect: Wounds

The features of entrance bullet wounds are different because they depend on several variable factors. Among the factors pertaining to the projectile itself are its velocity, its position at the moment of impact with the target and its size and shape. A high-velocity bullet will cause disproportionately greater damge compared to a low-velocity projectile. The other important factor is the density of the tissue. The greater the density of the tissue struck, the greater will be the damage. That is why bullets passing through soft tissues cause relatively slight damage and those hitting bones produce extensive injuries. Hollow organs filled with fluid, such as the heart, urine-filled bladder and the ventricles of the brain show great destruction because of hydrostatic forces. The passage of a bullet in such areas displaces the fluid in different directions and the forces of displaced fluid cause extensive lacerations.

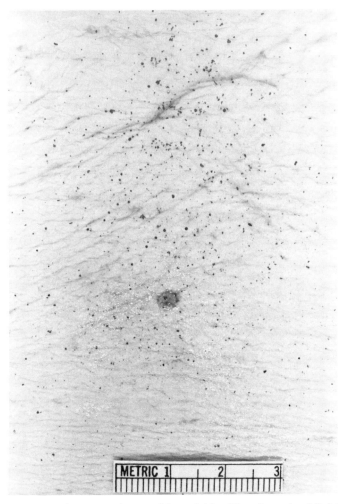

Fig. 8-11. A gunshot wound caused by a 0.22 caliber Saturday Night Special from a distance of 6 inches.

The mechanism of causation of bullet holes in the skin is simple. When the bullet strikes the skin, it pushes the skin so much that it is stretched to a point of rupture. The bullet enters the body through the rupture. Since the rifling of the gun imparts rotational motion to the bullet, it not only makes the hole round, but because the rotating bullet rubs against the stretched margins of the hole, it causes a rim of abrasion in the margins of the wound (Fig. 8-12). While the bullet is passing through the defect created by its nose, the diameter of the wound is greater than the diameter of the bullet. However, after the bullet leaves

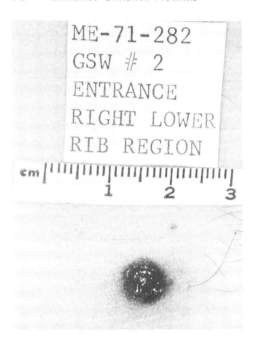

Fig. 8-12. Entrance gunshot wound showing a rim of abrasion in the margins.

the skin and enters deeper tissues the elasticity of the skin causes the wound to shrink. Then the wound has a diameter smaller than the diameter of the bullet.

The entrance gunshot wound is usually round if the bullet strikes the skin perpendicularly (Fig. 8-13). If there is thick bone immediately

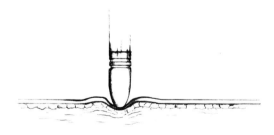

Fig. 8-13. Diagram illustrating a round wound caused by perpendicular strike of the bullet.

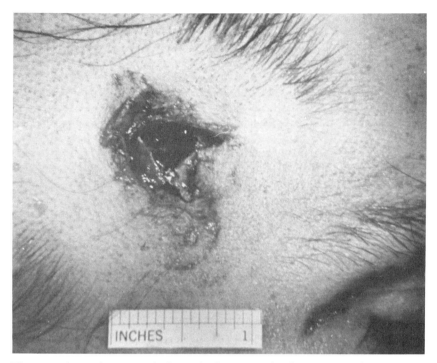

Fig. 8-14. A gunshot wound of temple showing subsidiary tears in the margins.

under the skin, the wound may not be round even with a perpendicular strike. The underlying bone resists the entry of gases, which blow back and cause subsidiary tears in the wound margins (Fig. 8-14). With a perfectly perpendicular strike, a rim of abrasion of uniform width is invariably seen in the entire margin of the wound. If, however, the bullet strikes the body at an angle, the gunshot wound may be round or oval, but the configuration of the abrasion is different. The first contact of the bullet causes an area of abrasion, and then the bullet enters the skin, causing the wound (Fig. 8-15). Such an abrasion on one side of the wound is a useful indicator of the direction of fire. The area of abrasion is always on the side of the wound nearest to the gun (Fig. 8-16).

Frequently, entrance gunshot wounds reveal grayish staining of the margins of the wound by grease (Fig. 8-17). This staining is caused by lubricant from the barrel of the gun and on the surface of the bullet. When the bullet enters the skin, the lubricant on the surface of the bullet is wiped off by the margins of the wound. Such a ring of grease staining in the margin of an entrance gunshot wound is called *ring of dirt* or *grease ring* or simply *grease mark*. This grease staining should not be interpreted as blackening of the skin from flame, smoke or gunpow-

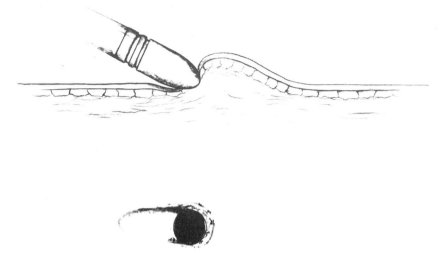

Fig. 8-15. A wound with abrasion on one side caused by angled strike of the bullet.

der. Such staining is commonly seen in wounds inflicted from long ranges. Grease rings are more prominent with lead bullets than with jacketed bullets.

Sometimes bullets strike the body at such an angle that they do not

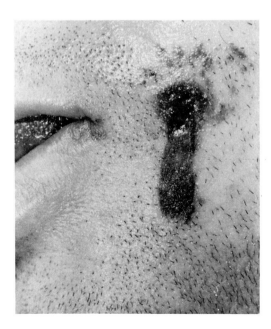

Fig. 8-16. An abrasion in the lower margin of gunshot wound caused by angled strike of the bullet.

Fig. 8-17. A gunshot wound
showing a grease mark in the
margins.

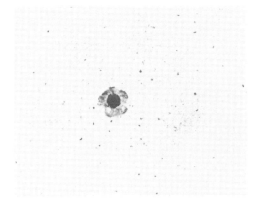

enter the tissues. They simply graze the skin and subcutaneous tissues,
causing a superficial abrasion or a laceration. Such an injury is called
bullet slap or *bullet graze* (Fig. 8-18). The injury is usually elongated or
oval and blackish-brown in color due to the effect of heat. If the bullet
causes an open deep track uniting the entrance and exit wounds in the
skin and subcutaneous tissues, the wound is called *gutter wound* (Fig.
8-19).

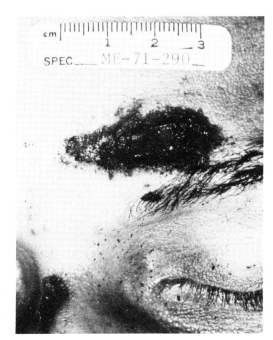

Fig. 8-18. A laceration-like
gunshot wound (bullet slap)
caused by grazing (glancing)
bullet.

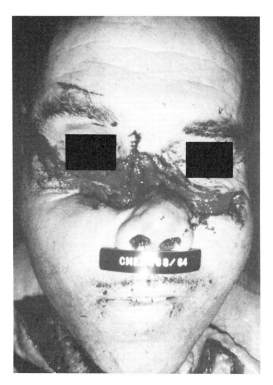

Fig. 8-19. A "gutter" gun-shot wound.

Metal Effect: Fouling

In addition to the features caused by the bullet, gunpowder, smoke and flame, occasionally one may find small fragments of metal embedded in the skin in the vicinity of the gunshot wound. The source of these particles is either the interior of the barrel of the gun or the bullet itself. When the bullet travels out of the barrel, it is rotated by lands and grooves within the barrel. If such a bullet fits tightly in the barrel, it tends to scrape the lands. Fragments of metal from the lands are ejected from the barrel and strike the target. On its way out from the barrel, the bullet itself may be damaged by the rifling of the gun and the fragments derived from it may similarly strike the target and be embedded in it (Fig. 8-20). Such metal fragments from the barrel or the bullet are found only when the range of fire is short. If the fragments of metal are stopped by intervening clothing one may only see small abrasions or superficial lacerations in the skin around the main wound. The finding of such fragments in the clothing will readily explain the causation of such injuries. Therefore, one must carefully examine the clothing for such fragments.

Fig. 8-20. The ear shows
metal fouling.

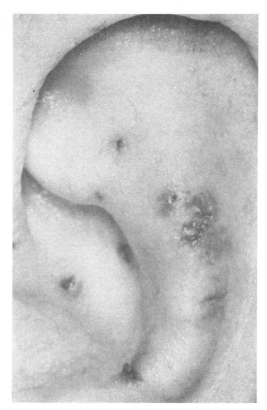

Muzzle Effect: Imprints of Muzzle

Sometimes the margins of an entrance gunshot wound in the skin or
the margins of a bullet hole in the clothing show the imprint of the
muzzle. Such a muzzle impression is caused when the gun is held in
contact with the clothing or with the skin (Fig. 8-21). The imprint is
considered by some to be the result of simple continuous pressure of
the muzzle on the skin. This is not the only explanation, however.
When the shot is fired, gases blow into and under the skin. These gases
blast the skin momentarily outwards causing it to strike against the
muzzle. This is the cause of muzzle imprinting in most instances.
Another factor may be at work. A gun that is held against the body may
be pushed momentarily away from the skin when the shot is fired.
Then it hits the body again because of continuous inward pressure and
the muzzle causes the imprint. If a single-barrel gun is used, the imprint of the firing muzzle may be seen around the margin of the wound.
With double-barrelled guns, one or both barrels may leave the imprint.
The nonfiring muzzle usually leaves the imprint in the form of a circular

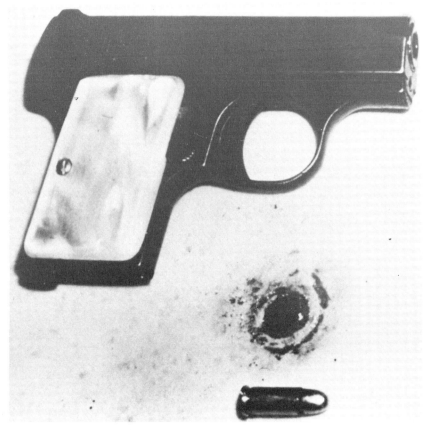

Fig. 8-21.   A gunshot wound showing the imprint of the muzzle.

abrasion corresponding in size to the muzzle (Fig. 8-22). In addition to the muzzle imprints, one may also see imprints caused by the attachments on the muzzle (Fig. 8-23).

Entrance Wounds in Bones

The bullet injuries in bones are often associated with features that can help differentiate entrance wounds from exit wounds. If the shot is fired with the muzzle in contact with the target or at close range, the bone may show flame effect and gunpowder blackening in the margins of the entrance wound. As in soft tissues, the exit holes are larger than the entrance defects. The passage of the bullet displaces the fragments of bone in the direction it travels, and hence it may be possible to identify the entrance defect in the bone from the direction of bone fragments. Entrance gunshot wounds in the skull are easy to differentiate from

Fig. 8-22. A contact shotgun wound with a circular abrasion (to the left of it) caused by the nonfiring muzzle.

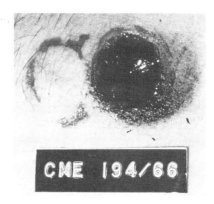

exit wounds. The skull is formed of an outer and an inner table. When the bullet enters the outer table, it causes a round entrance wound. When the same bullet exits from the inner table to enter the cranial cavity, there is bevelling, and the exit hole in the inner table is much larger than the hole in the outer table. If the bullet exits from the cranium, it causes a smaller hole in the inner table and a larger one in the outer table (Fig. 8-24).

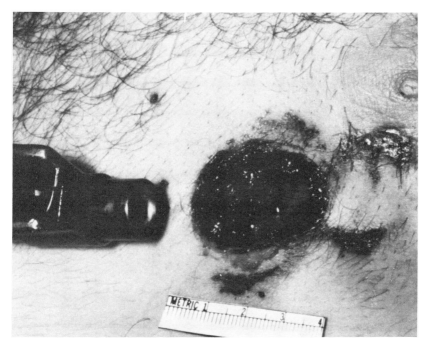

Fig. 8-23. A gunshot wound associated with an abrasion caused by the attachment of the muzzle.

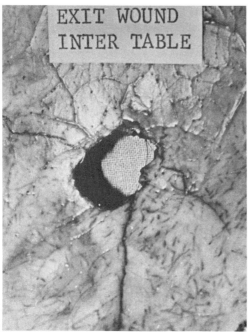

Fig. 8-24. (*Top*) A bullet hole in the skull. (*Bottom*) A bullet hole in the skull.

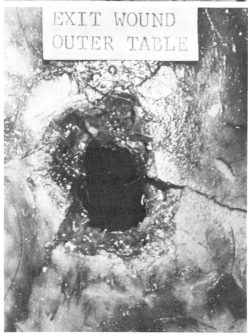

Re-entry Wounds

Re-entry wounds are not always easy to identify simply from external examination. Their features usually resemble those of wounds caused by long range fire. Of course, smoke smudging, gunpowder tattooing, flame burns and even grease marks are absent. The margins of the wounds usually show abrasion. Microscopic examination is usually not helpful (see below). The best way to identify the re-entry wounds is to line-up the entrance wounds with exit wounds and the bullets in the body (see Fig. 6-4).

CLASSIFICATION OF ENTRANCE GUNSHOT WOUNDS

The most important question in the cases of firearm injuries relates to the muzzle-target distance. Hence the entrance gunshot wounds in the skin are best classified on the basis of the range of fire. Depending on the distance of fire, the wounds can be classified into three categories: contact wounds, close-range wounds and long-range wounds. Alternatively, the wounds may be classified as hard-contact, soft-contact, near-shot and far-shot wounds. The characteristics of wounds of entry caused by pistols, revolvers and rifles are for the most part alike. Specific features of wounds caused by rifled weapons from various distances are described first. This will be followed by details of wounds caused by shotguns.

Contact Gunshot Wounds

A contact wound results when the muzzle of the firearm is pressed against the skin and the shot is fired. Such a wound is circular unless the shot is fired with the gun held at an angle. There is usually a thin band of contusion in the margins of the wound. In the contused area the hair is singed in many cases. In addition to the contusion, the margins of the perforation show burning caused by the flame. The charring by the flame causes dehydration and toughening of the margins as described above. The area immediately around the perforation is abraded, and this thin rim of abrasion is frequently covered with powder residue. Tattooing is minimal or absent. If the gun is held tightly against the skin, no gunpowder residue may be seen on the external surface of the wound (Fig. 8-25). In such instances gunpowder residue is present within the subcutaneous tissues and in the bullet track. If there is bone immediately under the skin, gunpowder blackening is frequently seen on the surface of the bone around the bullet hole. Also, contact wounds

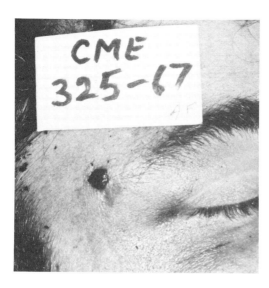

Fig. 8-25. A gunshot wound caused by a gun held tightly in contact with the skin. Note the absence of blackening of the margins.

in areas where there is bone immediately under the skin present variable shapes. Occasionally the margins of the wound of entry and the subcutaneous tissues show pinkish-red discoloration. This is due to formation of carboxyhemoglobin because of the presence of carbon monoxide in the gases in the shot blast.

Close-Range Wounds

Close-range wounds inflicted when the muzzle is in loose contact with the skin or from a distance of less than 24 inches have fairly typical characteristics. Helpful features consist of smoke and flame effect and tattooing. The flame effect occurs if the distance of fire is no more than 6 inches, and smoke smudging is seen frequently with distances of up to 12 inches. Tattooing by unburned gunpowder particles is seen around the entrance wound if the gun is fired from a distance of less than 24 inches (Fig. 8-26). Within this range, as the distance between the muzzle and the target increases, the area of scatter of unburned gunpowder becomes larger. Metal fouling is also seen sometimes with close-range gunshot wounds. Different guns of the same caliber and different ammunitions produce different patterns. Therefore, test fires are of utmost value in obtaining patterns of close-range wounds.

Long-Range Wounds

Long-range wounds caused by rifled weapons are usually round or oval with no blackening of the margins of the wounds by flame, smoke or gunpowder and no tattooing around them. Such wounds result when

Fig. 8-26. A close-range gunshot wound showing gunpowder stippling.

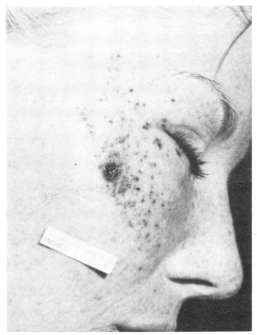

the range of fire is greater than 2 to 2½ feet. All wounds caused by civilian murder weapons in common use from distances over 2 to 2½ feet present more or less similar appearances. The only component of the shot involved in causing such wounds is the missile. The margins of the wounds commonly show, as has been already mentioned, a rim of abrasion and grease staining. There may also be a faint reddish discoloration of the margins of the perforation due to ecchymosis resulting from hemorrhage within the skin.

Entrance Shotgun Wounds

The components of a shotgun blast that cause various effects are the gunpowder, flame, smoke, gases, pellets and wads. The terms used to describe the effects of these shot components are the same as for rifled weapons.

The characteristics of shotgun injuries vary with the gauge of the weapon, degree of choke and the size and number of pellets. However, the nature of the entrance wounds caused by a shotgun depends to a great extent on the range of fire. Therefore, various characteristics of wounds are divided on the basis of range of fire.

Contact Wounds caused by shotguns with the muzzle pressed against

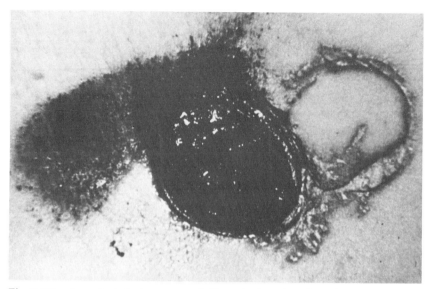

Fig. 8-27. A contact shotgun wound. Note the imprint of nonfiring muzzle and the blackening from the escape of gases.

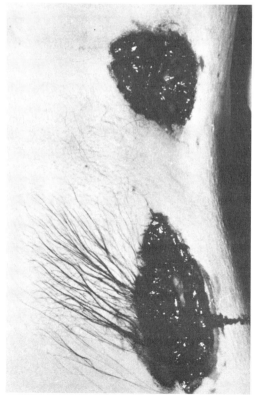

Fig. 8-28. Shotgun wounds in the axilla showing crenations in the margins caused by scattering pellets (cookie cutter etching).

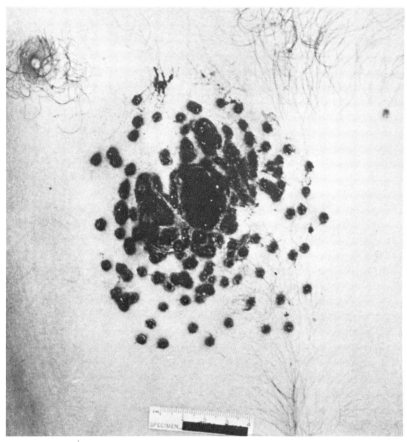

Fig. 8-29. Shotgun wound showing scatter of pellets.

the body of the decedent are usually round or oval. With a perpendicular position of the muzzle on the skin, the wound will be round. If the muzzle is held at an angle, the defect will be oval, and escape of gases may be obvious (Fig. 8-27). The margins of the wounds in the skin are usually clean cut, rarely ragged, and they show contusion of the tissue that is blackened by gunpowder. There may be singeing of the margins by flame associated with the shot. Because the shot and the gases are blasted within the wound, the subcutaneous and deeper tissues show severe disruption. With gases entering the body, the blood and the tissues along the track of the shot show the presence of carbon monoxide.

Close-Range Wounds caused when the muzzle is up to 24 inches from the body, but not pressed against the skin, depict certain identifiable characteristics. With a loose contact or with the muzzle up to 6 inches from the body, the wound is usually round or oval. The margins

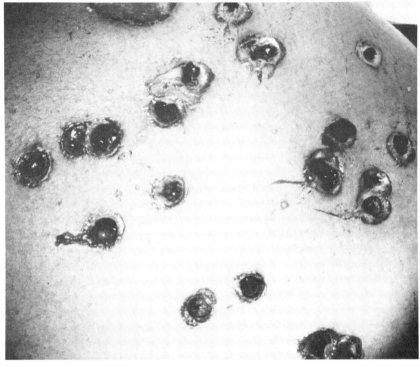

Fig. 8-30.   Pellet wounds showing rims of abrasion.

of the skin wound may be clean-cut or slightly ragged. There is some burning effect from the flame and blackening of the skin from smoke and unburned powder. The width of the zone of blackening increases with the increase in the distance of fire. Blackening due to smoke may be seen with ranges up to 15 inches. Tattooing by unburned powder may be seen in wounds caused by shotguns with the muzzle distance of up to 24 inches. The deeper tissues show marked disruption and may show the presence of carbon monoxide.

   Long-Range Wounds are defined for the purpose of present discussion as wounds caused by shotguns from a distance of over 24 inches. Although a wound caused from a distance of 2 to 3 feet may be a single round hole, with increasing range of fire the pellets start to scatter and cause subsidiary pellet holes. From a distance of 3 to 9 feet (1 to 3 yards) the shotgun produces a single large wound with crenations of the margins caused by the scattering pellets (Fig. 8-28). Longer distances reveal a greater scatter of pellets, causing small wounds around the main wound (Fig. 8-29). Individual pellet wounds are usually round and show a rim of abrasion at their margins (Fig. 8-30). From the degree of

Fig. 8-31. An x-ray showing widespread scatter of pellets within the body in a case of contact shotgun wound of chest-billiard ball ricochet effect (Courtesy of G. T. Mann, M.D.).

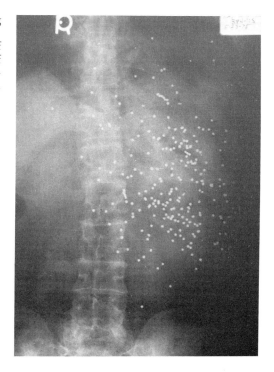

scatter of pellets, a rough estimate of the range of fire can be made. To make such an estimate, measure the distance between the two farthest pellets in inches and subtract one. The number thus obtained gives the range of fire in yards. This formula is applicable only if the barrel of the gun is unchoked. With a choke, the spread of the pellets is over a smaller area.

Although it is possible to make a rough estimate of the range of fire from the scatter of pellets when they hit the body, no attempt should be made to draw any conclusions about the range of fire from the scatter of pellets within the body. If a shot is fired from contact or close range and the pellets hit the body en masse, there is a tremendous dispersion of pellets within the body. This is because the pellets get deflected through stiking one another during their entry into the body.[3,4] This ricochet phenomenon has been termed the "billiard ball ricochet effect." This phenomenon may lead to erroneous conclusions about the range of fire if the shot pattern in the skin is obliterated because of decomposition or burning of the body and opinion is formed on the basis of scatter of pellets within the body as seen on x-rays.

A 59-year-old, white male who had been depressed for two weeks because he was convicted on an aggravated assault charge shot himself in the chest with a

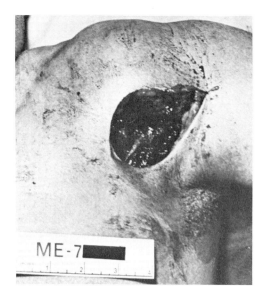

Fig. 8-32. A shotgun wound resembling a stab wound.

shotgun. He was lying on his back and the 28-gauge shotgun was lying near by. The shotgun wound measured 5/8 inch in diameter and there was a halo of blackening around the wound in an area 2 x 1½ inches. Although this was a contact shotgun wound, the scatter of pellets seen in the x-ray was over a large area (Fig. 8-31).

Not all shotgun wounds have a similar appearance. A shotgun wound may resemble a large stab wound (Fig. 8-32). If the shotgun is held against the body, gases are blasted into the body with the shot. Rapid entry of the shot and the gases causes a momentary vacuum immediately below the skin. This may result in the extrusion of soft tissues, such as fat, through the wound (Fig. 8-33). In addition to the wound caused by the shot, other injuries caused by wadding may be present.[6] The wadding is bulky but light. The wads do not travel as far as the pellets and do not have the same penetration capability. When they strike the body, therefore, they cause abrasions that are frequently circular (Fig. 8-34). The interposition of heavy clothing may alter the appearance of skin wounds. If the shot passes through clothing, the defects in the clothes, the pellet holes, and the presence or absence of blackening should be described.

CONCEALED ENTRANCE GUNSHOT WOUNDS

Gunshot wounds may not always be obvious and they may not have distinctive characteristics. If the body is covered with blood, the blood

Fig. 8-33. Protrusion of fat from a gunshot wound.

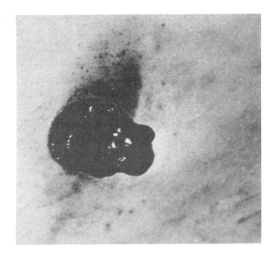

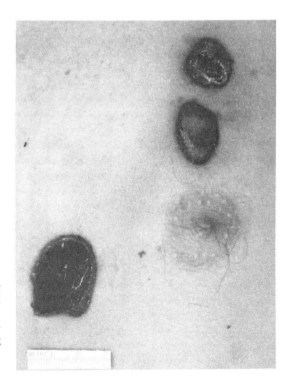

Fig. 8-34. A gunshot wound caused by rifled shotgun slug. The abrasions above the nipple were caused by wadding (Courtesy of J. E. Embry, M.D.).

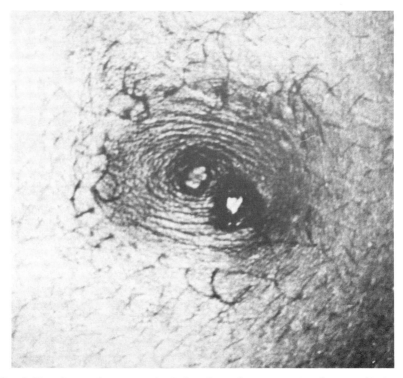

Fig. 8-35. A gunshot wound of the chest that was missed on preliminary external examination.

clots may obscure the firearm injury. In a case with multiple gunshot wounds, one entrance wound in the chest was missed on a preliminary external examination. X-rays and the finding of one too many bullets led to further search and the discovery of the wound (Fig. 8-35). In another case in which the body bore multiple gunshot wounds, the umbilicus was filled with blood. When this was cleaned away an additional gunshot wound was found within the umbilicus (Fig. 8-36).

Wounds in the head on which there is a thick growth of hair are not easily seen. A careful search must be made, and for proper examination of the wounds, the pathologist should not hesitate to shave the hair. Reflection of the scalp and opening of the cranium will reveal the bullet injury if the missile has entered the cranium.

The possibility of wounds in concealed sites should always be kept in mind.

Wounds in the mouth are not uncommon, most of these wounds being suicidal. A case of homicidal gunshot wound in the mouth has been reported.[5] This case and two other cases of homicidal gunshot

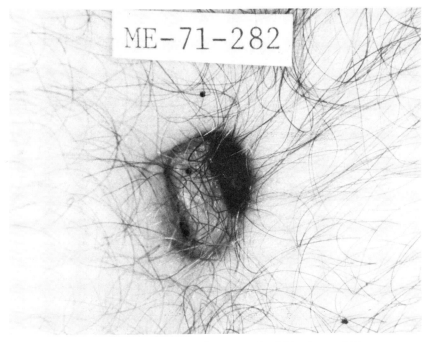

Fig. 8-36. An entrance gunshot wound within the umbilicus.

wounds of the mouth are discussed in Chapter 11. Wounds in the mouth are difficult to examine, especially if rigor has set in with the mouth closed. No effort should be spared, however, to explore such wounds. A mouth gag serves a useful purpose in such circumstances.

A wound in the nostril (Fig. 8-37) or one in the ear may escape detection if due care is not exercised at postmortem examination. A wound in the eye or in any of the body orifices, such as the rectum or vagina, may not be obvious. Therefore, the examiner must always look for bullet holes in the body orifices, axillae, perineum and back before and after the body is cleaned.

SPECIAL PROCEDURES TO IDENTIFY ENTRANCE GUNSHOT WOUNDS

Microscopic Appearances of Entrance Gunshot Wounds

Microscopic and chemical examinations and radiological techniques may be used to identify entrance gunshot wounds. Various components of a shot not only cause gross changes that have been described, but they also cause microscopic changes in the skin. The changes are mainly

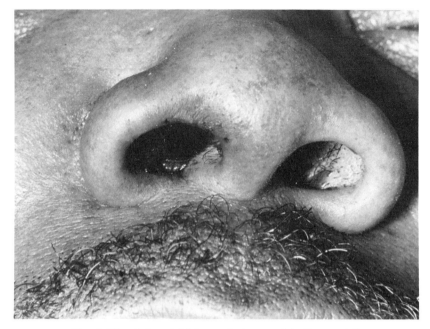

Fig. 8-37. A homicidal gunshot wound in the nostril.

caused by heat and mechanical trauma. The changes described here are not always constant, and they vary from case to case.

In contact and close-range wounds, one of the changes commonly seen is compression of the epithelium. Around the bullet hole a junction of normal epithelium and compressed epithelium can be seen. In the areas closer to the margin of the bullet hole progressively greater compression of the epithelium is evident. Elongation and flattening of epidermal cells with elongation of nuclei are seen. The epidermal cells within the margin of the perforation itself are distorted, disorganized or lost and may be mixed with gunpowder. Coagulation necrosis of the epithelium and swelling and vacuolization of the basal cells may also be present.[1] These epidermal changes are less prominent in long-range wounds. The abrading of the epidermis in the margin of the wound is a fairly constant feature of long-range wounds. The heat of the shot causes collagen changes. The collagen fibers may fuse, and they may show basophilic staining with hemotoxylin and eosin. Prominent features in the dermis are fresh hemorrhage and gunpowder residue. The cells in the dermis and the skin appendages may show shrinking of nuclei, vacuolization and pyknosis.

The presence of gunpowder particles in the entrance wounds is helpful in differentiating these wounds from the exit wounds. The powder residue may also help in making an estimate of the range of fire. The gunpowder particles are seen as black or blackish-brown clumps of amorphous material. They may be on the skin, in the epidermis and dermis or in the subcutaneous and deep tissues. With a tight contact, the skin surface around the wound usually shows very little or no gunpowder whereas the subcutaneous tissues show considerable amounts. There is some gunpowder residue on the surface of the skin if the wound is caused with the gun held loosely against the skin. Skin layers and subcutaneous tissues also show gunpowder particles in such wounds. In close-range wounds, deposits of powder are prominently seen on the surface of the skin with variable amounts in the skin layers. The only gunpowder in long-range wounds is carried by the bullet. Hence minimal gunpowder is seen in such wounds.

A special histological technique for forensic ballistics has been described by Rolfe and his colleagues.[7]

Chemical Identification of Entrance Gunshot Wounds

Several chemical entities get deposited on the clothing and on the skin (in and around the entrance gunshot wound) when a shot is fired. The smokeless gunpowder residue leaves detectable nitrites and cellulose nitrates on the area struck. If black gunpowder is used, potassium, carbon, nitrites, nitrates, sulphides, sulphates, carbonates, thiocyanates and thiosulphates may be deposited on the clothing and the skin. The primer residue in modern weapons contains lead and barium. In addition, antimony, mercury and other components may be found in the primer residue. Walker analyzed 96 primer residues and found the following elements in percentages indicated.[8]

Element	*Percentage of Primer Residue*
Barium	90 per cent
Antimony	87 per cent
Lead	75 per cent
Mercury	67 per cent
Potassium	31 per cent
Tin	9 per cent
Manganese	4 per cent

Also ejected may be rust from the gun barrel and lead, antimony, tin, nickel, copper, bismuth, silver and thallium from the bullets and a number of elements fouling the gun barrel.

The detection of some of these elements in the clothes or in the skin together with consideration of other aspects of the case will help in identifying a wound as an entrance wound.

Radiological Identification of Entrance Gunshot Wounds

The radiology techniques that can be used to identify entrance gunshot wounds are discussed in Chapter 7.

EFFECT OF INTERPOSITION OF CLOTHING ON ENTRANCE GUNSHOT WOUNDS

While interpreting the entrance gunshot wounds, one must bear in mind the possible effect of intervening clothing. The thickness of the clothing, the nature of the fabric and the number of layers of the garment can alter the appearances of the entrance gunshot wounds in the skin.

The examination of the clothing should first be undertaken to determine the number of bullet holes and to identify the holes caused by entering bullets. The holes caused by bullets fired from contact and close ranges will show the effect of smoke, flame and gunpowder. In a case of long-range fire, the clothing may show only grease marks.

If the bullet perforates the clothing before it enters the skin, the effect of smoke, flame and gunpowder may be less pronounced on the skin. A single layer of thin clothing may not make much difference, but thick fabric or multiple layers may stop the smoke and gunpowder particles, and the underlying skin wounds may be devoid of features of contact or close-range wounds. The clothing may also stop metal fragments. The metal fragments hitting the body will cause trivial abrasions and they may be found trapped in the intervening fabric instead of being embedded in the skin. In cases of long-range fire, the grease mark or dirt ring in the margins of the skin wound may be less pronounced or absent if the grease on the bullet is wiped off by the intervening clothing.

Sometimes the passage of a bullet through the clothing will help identify the wound in the skin as an entrance wound if fibers of clothing carried by the shot blast are found within the skin wound.

REFERENCES

1. Adelson, L.: A microscopic study of dermal wounds. Am. J. Clin. Pathol., 35:393, 1961.
2. ———.: The Pathology of Homicide. Charles C Thomas, Springfield, Illinois, 1974.
3. Breitenecker, R.: Shotgun wound patterns. Am. J. Clin. Pathol., 52:258, 1969.
4. Breitenecker, R. and Senior, W.: Shotgun patterns. I. An experimental study on the influence of intermediate targets. J. For. Sci., 12:193, 1967.

5. Fatteh, A.: Homicidal gunshot wound of mouth. J. Forensic Sci. Soc., 12:347, 1972.
6. Guerin, P. F.: Shotgun wounds, J. Forensic Sci., 5:294, 1960.
7. Rolfe, H. C., Curle, D., and Simmons, D.: A histological technique for forensic ballistics. J. Forensic Med., 18:47, 1971.
8. Walker, J. T.: Bullet holes and chemical residues in shooting cases. J. Crim. Law and Criminol., 31:497, 1940.

9

Exit Gunshot Wounds

The examination of exit gunshot wounds can provide useful information. In order to be able to lead to any conclusions, the wounds must first be properly identified; the examiner must attempt to establish that the wound he is examining is caused by a firearm and that it is an exit wound and not an entrance wound. In view of the fact that the exit gunshot wounds may resemble perforating injuries caused by pointed objects and may mimic lacerations and at times incised wounds, it may not be possible to identify them as exit gunshot wounds unless corroborative evidence is analyzed. The history of shooting, features of the entrance wound, finding of a spent bullet or cartridge case and the internal examination of the body will aid in identifying an exit wound. In some instances, the entrance and exit wound may look alike. It is obviously important to distinguish one from the other. All available information must be considered, and the entrance and the exit wounds examined in light of such information before drawing a conclusion about whether a wound is an entrance or an exit wound.

In what ways can the examination of an exit wound help? The exit wound can help determine (1) the direction of fire; (2) the posture of the victim at the time of the shooting; and (3) the number of missiles in the body. The location of an exit wound in relation to an entrance wound will serve as a reliable means in most cases to determine the direction of fire. The investigator should, however, bear in mind the possibility of deflection of the bullet during its course through the body. As has been pointed out in the previous chapter the lining up of the entrance wound, bullet track and the exit wound or the lining up of the entrance wound, exit wound, re-entry wound and the re-exit wound will assist in determining not only the direction of fire but also, in some instances, the posture of the victim at the time of the shooting. The presence of exit wounds in a case of shooting will indicate to the examiner the number of bullets in the body. An equal number of entrance and exit wounds generally suggests exit of all missiles, whereas fewer exit holes

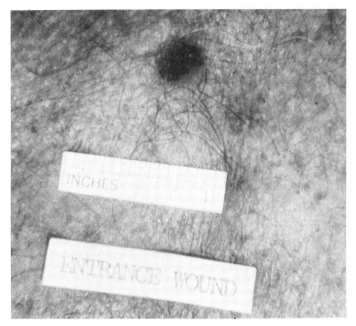

Fig. 9-1. Small entrance wound caused by AR-15 semiautomatic rifle.

will indicate the number of bullets still in the body. Exit holes caused by fragments of bullets, bones, or both can cause misinterpretation unless they are correctly identified.

FEATURES OF EXIT WOUNDS

Exit wounds in the skin are caused the same way as entrance wounds. The only difference in exit wounds is that the stretching force of the bullet that perforates the skin is from inside out. In most instances, most defects are caused only by the bullets or pellets. Such other components of the shot as flames, smoke, gunpowder and even wadding that cause characteristic features at the site of entry do not play any part in imparting any features to exit wounds unless the shot passes through a small mass of soft tissues, as in the extremities.

Exit wounds can be difficult to interpret because they vary in size and shape. The *size of the exit wound* varies because of several factors. These are:

1. Velocity of the bullet at the point of exit
2. Surface area of the bullet striking the point of exit
3. Deformation of the missile
4. Yawing and tumbling of the bullet

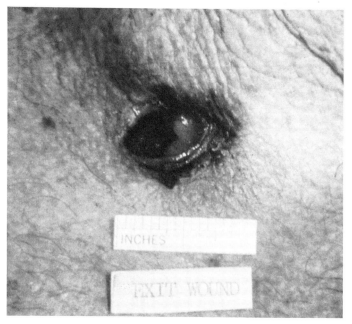

Fig. 9-2.   Large exit wound caused by AR-15 semiautomatic rifle.

5. Fragmentation of the bullet
6. Presence or absence of fragments of bone accompanying the bullet through the exit wound
7. Presence or absence of bone under the skin in the area of exit
8. Presence or absence of objects pressing against the skin in the area of exit

The *velocity of the bullet* and its size are important factors in relation to the size of the wound that it causes. The ability of a bullet to cause a wound is directly proportional to its size and directly proportional to the square of its velocity. Therefore, with increasing velocity the tissue damage is disproportionately greater. The greater the velocity of the bullet at the point of exit, the larger will be the exit hole. The following case report illustrates this well:

A 58-year-old white male, while attempting to hold up a grocery store, was shot by the store manager with his high velocity (3150 feet per second) AR-15 semi-automatic rifle. One shot entered the back of the head. The entrance wound measured only 1/16-inch in diameter. The passage of the bullet, 0.223 caliber, through the cranium exploded it, shattering almost the whole skull into many fragments. A second shot entered the back of the right side of the neck (Fig. 9-1). The entrance wound measured 1/16 inch in diameter. The bullet traversed soft tissue, and when it exited on the front of the neck it caused a much larger exit wound measuring ½ inch in diameter (Fig. 9-2).

An intact bullet will cause a gunshot wound in proportion to its size, but if the same bullet has a larger striking surface it will cause a proportionately larger exit wound. The increase in the *area of striking surface of the bullet* results from deformation of the bullet while it is passing through the body. Some bullets, for instance, become mushroomed at their nose ends while they pass through the tissue. Passage through a bone invariably results in deformation of the bullet. Such deformities cause an increase in the surface of the bullet that strikes the tissue at the point of exit. The result is an exit wound larger than the entrance wound.

Even if the bullet is not deformed during its course through the body, it may cause an exit hole larger than the entrance hole. This may occur due to the *yawing or tumbling* of the bullet. A bullet travelling in an irregular fashion instead of travelling nose on is called a yawing bullet, and one that rotates end-on-end during its motion is called a tumbling bullet. Such motions of the bullet may cause it to hit the area of exit obliquely or along the length of the bullet rather than nose on. The larger surface area of the side of the bullet striking the tissues at the exit will thus cause a larger exit hole than the smaller nose on striking surface of the bullet.

The increase in the area of the striking surface of a bullet at the point of exit due to deformation, yawing or tumbling explains why the *exit wounds are usually larger than the entrance wounds*. It must be remembered that at contact range the entrance wound may be larger than the exit wound because the gases in the shot blast contribute to the damage of the tissue, creating a larger entrance wound.

Fragmentation of a bullet will create exit holes of variable sizes. The main bulk of the bullet as well as the fragments may cause exit wounds. The largest piece will be smaller than the intact bullet, but deformation of the piece and irregularities in its motion will contribute to the uneven size of the exit wound.

At times, a bullet shatters a bone and exits with small fragments of bone. The fragments of bone accompanying the bullet will contribute to the tearing of the skin at the point of exit and enlargement of the exit wound. Even if the bone fragments do not exit, shattering of the bone may add to the tearing of tissues. This is particularly true for the head area. The damage to the outer table over a larger area (at the point of exit) than in the inner table may account for large exit wounds.

The presence of objects pressing against the skin in the area of exit of the bullet may affect the size of the exit hole. The pressure from such objects limits external stretching of the margins of the perforated skin. Consequently the subsidiary tears are not as extensive as they would otherwise be. The exit hole in such circumstances tends to be small and round with minimal tearing of the margins.

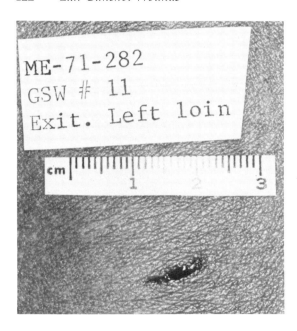

Fig. 9-3. An exit gunshot wound resembling a laceration.

Exit wounds may present themselves in different *shapes*. They may be round, stellate or cruciate. Sometimes, they are elliptical or crescent-shaped and occasionally they present as linear lacerations and even resemble incised wounds (Fig. 9-3). When a bullet passes only through

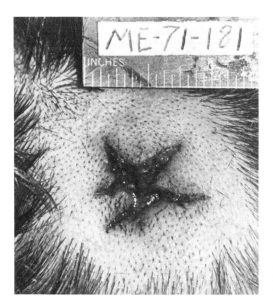

Fig. 9-4. Radial tears in the margins of an exit gunshot wound.

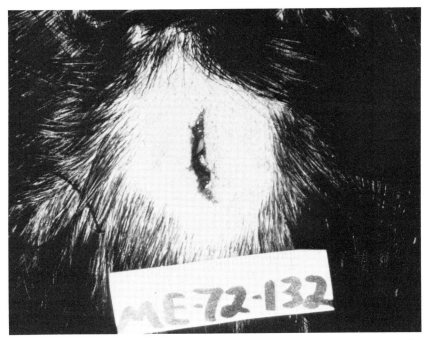

Fig. 9-5. An exit gunshot wound of head associated with fractures of skull.

soft tissues and exits, the exit hole may appear round. However, a careful examination of such a hole will reveal small subsidiary lacerations in the margins. The other circumstance in which the exit bullet hole may be round is when the bullet leaves the body against external resistance. A perfectly round exit wound with no tears in the margins is rare. In most instances, the tearing effect of the exiting bullet causes irregularly shaped exit wounds. Stellate exit wounds are more often seen in the head. In the head region, the exiting bullet perforates the skull and fractures it. The energy spread is in a radial fashion, and this is responsible for radial tears in the margins of an exit wound, giving it a stellate appearance (Fig. 9-4). Fractures of the skull may result in uneven exertion of outward force, giving a variety of other shapes to exit wounds (Fig. 9-5).

Other features that are helpful in identifying the exit wounds are eversion of the margins of the wounds and protrusion of tissue tags through the defect.

Exit Holes in Skull

The exit holes in the skull are always larger than the entrance holes. As has been explained in the previous chapter, the bullet entering the

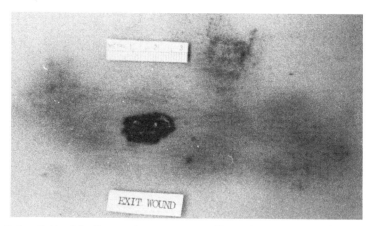

Fig. 9-6. Exit of bullet against pressure. Note the presence of contusions around the gunshot wound.

cranium causes bevelling of the inner table of the skull at the point of entry into the cranial cavity. When it leaves the cranium, it again causes bevelling of the outer table at the point of exit from the cranium. Thus, the exit hole in the inner table in the area of entry into the cranium is larger than the entrance hole in the outer table in that area. At the point of exit from the cranial cavity, the hole in the outer table is larger than the one in the inner table.

When the skull is shattered the exit hole may not be obvious. In some cases of a gunshot wound of the mouth, the top of the cranium is extensively fractured by the shot blast. A widely open top of the head represents the exit wound in such cases.

Exit of Bullet Against Pressure

If a bullet exits from the skin without any resistance other than the tissue resistance, an exit hole with subsidiary tears results. Such an exit wound is not associated with any obvious contusion of the tissue and does not usually show a rim of abrasion in the margin such as in the margin of an entrance wound. If, however, the bullet exits from the skin against pressure from a firm or hard object in contact with the skin, the appearances of the exit wounds are different. Under such circumstances there may be an obvious area of contusion of the skin around the bullet hole (Fig. 9-6). If the object in contact with the skin is hard and the bullet exits against considerable resistance from it, the exit wound may not only be round but it may show a rim of abrasion in its margins. Such exit wounds could easily be mistaken for entrance wounds. Exit wounds of this nature may be seen when the victim is lying on the ground or standing against a wall when shot and the exited bullet is stopped by the ground or the wall. They may also be caused when the exited bullet hits a belt, buckle, tough clothing or a similar object in tight contact with the skin.

Partly Exited Bullet (Partial Exit Wound)

A bullet that passes through parts of the body may stop short of exiting from the body. Because of the toughness and elasticity of the skin, bullets are frequently stopped in the subcutaneous tissues. Occasionally, a bullet makes a partial exit. This may be due to resistance offered by some firm or hard object in contact with the skin. In such an instance, the bullet that is stopped in the skin may cause an incomplete tear. Such a tear often resembles a small incised wound.

More Than One Exit Wound Per Entrance Wound

There are three circumstances under which one may see more exit wounds than entrance wounds. First, the bullet that enters the body, causing one entrance wound, may break up during its course within the body. Individual pieces of the bullet may leave the body, causing multiple exit wounds. The bullet may fragment in the body if it hits a bone or if there is some defect in the metal. Secondly, the bullet may fracture a bone in the body and the fragments of bone may be blasted out of the body causing additional wounds. Thirdly, two shots may be fired in succession at one point on the body, causing one entrance wound, but the two bullets may exit at separate points. It is also possible for two bullets to be fired at the same time, entering the body at one point but exiting separately.

Exit Gunshot Wounds in Decomposed Bodies

The interpretation of entrance and exit gunshot wounds is rendered difficult by decomposition of the body. The appearances of the wounds may be markedly altered. If there was continuous external pressure in the area of the exit wound, the injury may appear smaller than it was initially. On the other hand, pouring out of fluids from the body and protrusion of fat and visceral tissue such as a loop of intestine may enlarge the wound considerably. Not only the size and the shape of the wounds are modified but other identifying features may be obliterated.

Exit Shotgun Wounds

In a person shot with a shotgun, pellets may exit from the body if they pass superficially or if an extremity is struck. If exit wounds caused by pellets are present, they may help establish the direction of fire and reconstruct the posture of the victim at the time of shooting. The exit holes caused by pellets have variable appearances but generally they are

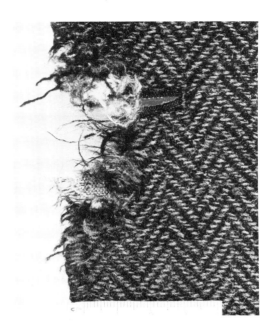

Fig. 9-7. Exit hole in fabric. Note the eversion of fibers.

round or oval and have everted margins. If the shotgun is loaded with slugs, the appearances of the exit wounds will be variable too.

HISTOPATHOLOGY OF EXIT WOUNDS

The pathological alterations in exit wounds are minimal or absent. The changes caused by heat in the epidermis are absent in most cases, since the bullet loses heat during its passage through the body. The skin may show collagen changes due to some remaining heat in the bullet. The epidermis does not usually show any epithelial alteration except disorganization of cells in the margins of the wound. There is usually some fresh hemorrhage in the epidermis and the dermis. The gunpowder residue is also absent unless the bullet has traversed only a short distance through the tissues, as in the wounds of extremities. If there is any powder residue in the area of an exit wound, it is usually in the dermal tissue.

EXIT HOLES IN CLOTHES

Exit holes in clothes caused by bullets do not provide as much useful information as do the entrance holes. The eversion of the margins of the defect may give some idea about the side of the material from which the bullet came out if it is not soiled by blood or fluids, folded, or otherwise tampered with (Fig. 9-7).

10

The Autopsy

The main purposes of a medicolegal autopsy are to determine the cause and manner of death, to collect evidence and to develop such ancillary matters as the identity of the deceased, characteristics of the fatal weapon and other matters that will help to solve the medicolegal questions that may arise. In this chapter the procedures vitally important in the investigation of deaths from gunshot wounds are discussed.

As in any other case, the pathologist about to perform an autopsy on the body of a shooting victim must bear in mind certain general principles. These are:

1. Authorization for an autopsy must be checked.
2. As much information as possible must be obtained before starting the autopsy.
3. All unauthorized persons must be excluded.
4. The examination of the body in the autopsy room must be complete. Even in straightforward cases, nothing should be left undone.
5. In the collection of materials of evidence, it is always better to collect too much rather than too little.
6. If it is necessary to call for assistance, the pathologist should not hesitate to do so.

Authorization for Autopsy

Any death resulting from firearm injuries is a medicolegal case. The authorization for an autopsy on a medicolegal case depends on the local law. In jurisdictions with medical examiner systems, duly appointed medical examiners or the Chief Medical Examiner can legally authorize an autopsy; where the coroner system is retained the Coroner signs the permit. Before commencing the autopsy, the pathologist must make sure that he has the authority to perform the autopsy. If the Coroner or the Medical Examiner has authorized an autopsy on a medicolegal case, objections from the members of the decedent's family should not be allowed to interfere with the pathologist's duties.

History of the Circumstances of Death

The pathologist must gather all the information about the circumstances of death prior to autopsy. Such information will guide him as to what procedure to follow in performing the autopsy and what specimens to collect. Lack of such information may result in failure to collect vital evidence.

Initial Steps in the Autopsy Room

The following procedures should form a part of the autopsy on a case of shooting, especially on a victim of homicide:
1. Photograph the remains in the condition received.
2. Collect articles of evidential value.
3. Describe the clothing.
4. Take x-rays of the body.
5. Take a photograph of the face with identifying number.
6. Record rectal temperature if indicated.
7. Obtain a sample of scalp hair by plucking tufts of hair with the hand or with clamps. (Do not cut the hair.)

COLLECTION OF TRACE EVIDENCE

Collection of trace evidence from the body is an important aspect of an autopsy. If the pathologist did not go to the scene of death, he should inquire about what materials have been taken from the body. The pathologist should then examine the body in the condition received with a view to determine if there are any traces of articles of evidential value. This is of importance because handling of the body may result in loss of some of these articles. After a review of this nature, the pathologist should proceed to collect the trace evidence. He should be particularly careful in collecting such evidence if the case is a homicide. Every piece of physical evidence should be placed in an appropriate container, and each container should be clearly labeled with the decedent's name, a description of the material, the name of the person collecting the evidence and the date it is collected. The chain of custody of all the materials collected, it must be stressed again, can be a vital issue at a trial. If the evidence is given to the police officer or any other investigator present at the autopsy, a written receipt should be obtained from him. If the material has to be mailed, it should be sent by registered mail with return receipt requested.

In cases of gunshot wounds particular attention should be paid to the collection of the following articles of evidence.

Blood Spots. There may be blood spots on the victim's clothing or on his body. This may be assailant's blood. In case of a struggle between the victim and the assailant, the assailant may get injured and his blood may be left on the victim's clothes or body. Collection of such blood and determination of its group may give a clue to the identity of the assailant.

Hairs and Fibers. Any time the victim and the assailant come in contact with each other there is always a possibility of exchange of traces of evidence. Any degree of struggle is likely to result in something from the assailant's body or clothes being left on the victim. The victim may attempt to hold on to the assailant by catching his clothing or hair. In such circumstances, fibers from the assailant's clothes or his hair may be found on the victim's body. It is important to retain a sample of the victim's scalp hair, for they may be required for comparison.

Nail Scrapings. Valuable evidence may on occasion be found under the victim's nails. The scrapings under the nails may reveal traces of fibers from the assailant's clothes, his hair, blood and even tissue (such as epidermis) if there was a struggle and if the victim attempted to push the assailant, hold on to him, ward off his attack or injure the assailant with his hands.

Gunshot Residue. Gunshot residue may be found in the areas of gunshot wounds on the victim or on the victim's hands. Partially burned or unburned particles of gunpowder and metallic components of the residue should be collected from these areas before such areas are washed or disturbed in any way. The components of the gunshot residue may be identified by chemical tests, neutron activation analysis or atomic absorption technique.

The so-called Paraffin Test for the detection of nitrites and nitrates in the gunpowder left on the hand of the person firing the gun, on the clothes and on the skin around the gunshot wounds is used in many places. The method of testing is simple. A paraffin glove is prepared by placing layers of melted paraffin on the victim's hand or by soaking a piece of gauze with melted paraffin and while still melted wrapping around the hand. After the paraffin is solidified the glove is removed and treated with diphenylamine or diphenylbenzidine reagent. The spots where nitrates, nitrites or other oxidizing agents are present will show blue discoloration. However, this test has limited value and, in fact, a critical study by Cowan and Purdon suggests that it is useless and should be abandoned.[1]

Another simple method of picking up gunshot residue is to swab the area with cotton swabs dipped in 5 per cent nitric acid solution. The National Office Laboratory of the U.S. Treasury Department recommends the following procedure to obtain such swabs:

1. Put on clean gloves.

2. Swab thoroughly the back of the victim's left hand and fingers with two separate single-ended cotton tipped swabs, each moistened with six drops of 5 per cent nitric acid. Place both swabs in a plastic vial and label the container with information about the area swabbed, case number, examiner's signature and the date.

3. Similarly, swab the palm of the left hand, palm of the right hand and the back of the right hand, each with two swabs moistened with 5 per cent nitric acid. Place each pair of swabs in a separate container and label the containers appropriately.

4. Also, place two swabs simply moistened with six drops of 5 per cent nitric acid in a container to serve as control.

These swabs can be sent to the National Office Laboratory—Alcohol, Tobacco and Firearms Division, Room 7575, 1111 Constitution Avenue, N.W., Washington, D.C., 20224—for testing by Neutron Activation Analysis (NAA). A letter giving the facts of the case such as case number, name of the person processed for gunshot residue, caliber and manufacturer of the ammunition, type of weapon and name of the agency requesting the examination must accompany the swabs.

The Neutron Activation Analysis can detect antimony and barium, whereas atomic absorption spectrophotometry can be used to make quantitative determination of lead. These techniques are described in detail in Chapter 17.

If the assailant is apprehended, the articles of trace evidence described above should be collected from his clothes and body just the same way as from the victim.

Handling of Clothing

The examination of clothing in a case of a gunshot wound fatality is important, especially if the clothes show bullet holes. The assistants in the autopsy room must be instructed not to undress the body in the absence of the pathologist. Before the body is disrobed, careful examination of the garments must be undertaken. All items of evidential value on the clothes should be photographed in place and their locations recorded by description before they are picked up. A careful search should then be made to find the bullet holes. Each bullet hole should be photographed and described. The description should include the location of the bullet hole, its dimensions and whether it shows flame, smoke, gunpowder or grease effect. If any of these effects are observed, measurements of the areas must be recorded. Occasionally, one may find tiny fragments of metal (broken off from the barrel or the bullet) stuck to the clothing. After the area bearing these fragments is photographed and described, the fragments should be picked up and retained. If the victim is shot through glass or a metal screen, fragments of these materials may also be found embedded in the clothing. Efforts should be made to differentiate entrance holes in the clothing from exit holes. Observations about the direction in which the fibers of the clothing around the bullet hole are pushed should be made. Notes indicating the relationship of the bullet holes in the clothing and the gunshot wounds on the body should be made. There may be more bullet holes in the clothing than on the body if the bullet passes through folded areas of the clothing.

Only after these preliminaries are completed should the body be undressed. The clothes should be removed intact and not cut or torn. As each garment is removed it should be listed with a note about its color and the nature of the fabric. If any loose bullet or bullet fragment is found while removing the clothes, it should be carefully picked up and preserved after noting the location where it is found.

If the clothes are wet, they should be dried before they are placed in bags. Care should be exercised while placing them in bags so as not to fold them in the areas of bullet holes. Carelessness in the handling of the clothes may result in the loss of some gunpowder particles, metallic fragments or other articles of evidence that may have been embedded in the clothing.

After the pathologist has completed his examination of the clothes, he may release them to the police for further examination. He must obtain a receipt for every item that he delivers to the police officer.

X-RAY EXAMINATION

It is advisable to x-ray the body of the victim of a gunshot wound prior to autopsy if facilities are available. Anterior and lateral films of the general area in which the bullet is suspected to be lodged save a considerable amount of the pathologist's time and effort in the search for the missile. In addition to the principal purpose of localizing the missiles, x-rays also help determine the number of bullets in the body, evaluate the direction and angle of fire, estimate the distance of fire, assess the depth of the wounds and determine the type of firearm.[2] These and other uses of x-rays are discussed in detail in Chapter 7.

X-rays of the body with the clothes on may include artefactual shadows of buttons, coins and other metallic objects. These may create confusion. Also, any bullets lying loose in the clothes may be included in the x-rays and be interpreted as being in the body, leading to unnecessary search. In order to avoid such situations, it is advisable to make x-rays of the body after it is undressed.

Since one of the important values of x-rays is that they form a permanent record for use in courts, each of the plates must be properly identified with the case number and the date of examination.

The pathologist should study the x-rays before he commences the internal examination of the body to determine the point of lodgement of the bullet.

PHOTOGRAPHIC DOCUMENTATION

The importance of photographic documentation of a case cannot be overemphasized. Color and black-and-white photographs will portray what words cannot adequately describe. Various aspects of photography in the autopsy are discussed in Chapter 6.

EXTERNAL EXAMINATION

The external examination in a medicolegal case is always important. Of particular importance are the aspects of identification and injuries. Other vital aspects related to external examination are the collection of specimens and the determination of the time of death. In view of the significance of the external examination, it is imperative that nothing be left undone in any shooting case.

General External Examination

The general description of the body should include the age, sex, race, color of skin, height, weight, nutrition, muscle development, body build, bony frame, congenital and acquired deformities, scars, tattoos, moles, skin diseases and the distribution, nature and color of hair. A note should be made of the presence and distribution of lividity (hypostasis), rigor mortis and signs of decomposition. The eyes should be examined for color, size of pupils and the presence or absence of petechial hemorrhages. The mouth should be carefully examined for teeth and dentures, especially in cases in which the dental record is important. In males, a note should be made about whether or not the penis is circumcised.

Examination of the external injuries other than the gunshot wounds should not be conducted lightly. Every effort should be made to record a verbal description, sketch the injuries on a body diagram and photograph them. The nature and the direction of abrasions, the color of bruises and the characteristics of lacerations and incised wounds should be noted with measurements. The back should always be examined for injuries.

Examination of Gunshot Wounds

The best way to document gunshot wounds, aside from photographing them, is to draw them on Body Diagrams (Fig. 10-1) and record the

BODY DIAGRAM—HEAD

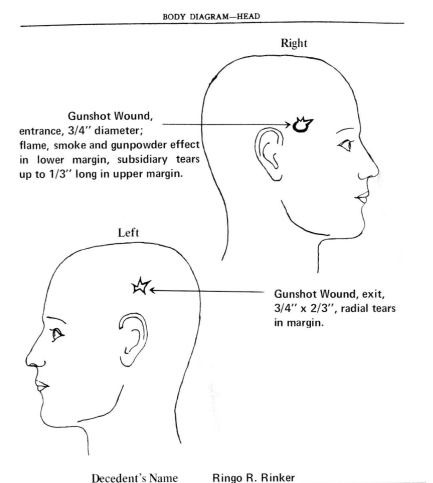

Right

Gunshot Wound, entrance, 3/4" diameter; flame, smoke and gunpowder effect in lower margin, subsidiary tears up to 1/3" long in upper margin.

Left

Gunshot Wound, exit, 3/4" x 2/3", radial tears in margin.

Decedent's Name ___ Ringo R. Rinker
Examined
By   Jerry J. Joshua, M.D.   Date Jan. 1, 1975

Fig. 10-1.   A method of documenting gunshot wounds; hypothetical data filled in.

details of the wounds on the Gunshot Wound Information Chart. Before these records are made, however, the entrance and exit wounds should be identified. If the gunshot wounds are in hairy areas, such as the scalp, the pathologist should not hesitate to shave the area so that the wounds can be examined and photographed.

If there are multiple gunshot wounds, they should be assigned numbers. These numbers will serve as good reference points. The wounds on the body may be numbered with an ink marker (Fig. 10-2) or a typed or hand written number may be placed next to the wound (Fig. 10-3).

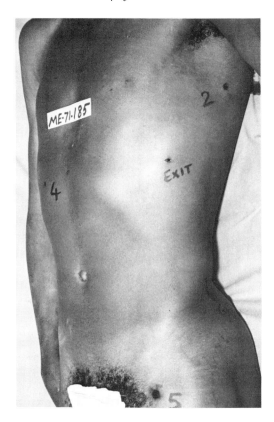

Fig. 10-2. Numbering of gunshot wounds with an ink marker will facilitate reference.

Photographs should first be taken with these numbers and identifying information.

On the *Body Diagrams* the wounds should be drawn as they appear on the body. The number assigned to the wound should be placed next to the diagram of the wound with a short description of the wound such as "Gunshot wound No. 1, entrance, round, ¼-inch in diameter, with a rim of abrasion ¹/₁₆-inch wide in the margins of the bullet hole," or "Gunshot wound No. 3, entrance, oval, ¼ × ¹/₅-inches, with gunpowder tattooing in an area 3 inches in diameter." The diagram of the wound on the body chart should depict the gunpowder tattooing or other features to correspond with the features on the body.

If any of the bullets is palpable under the skin, its location should be marked on the body diagram with a note such as "Bullet palpable under skin, 26 inches from the top of the head and 4 inches to the left of midline."

The *Gunshot Wound Information Chart,* if properly completed, will indicate the location of the gunshot wound on the body, its dimensions

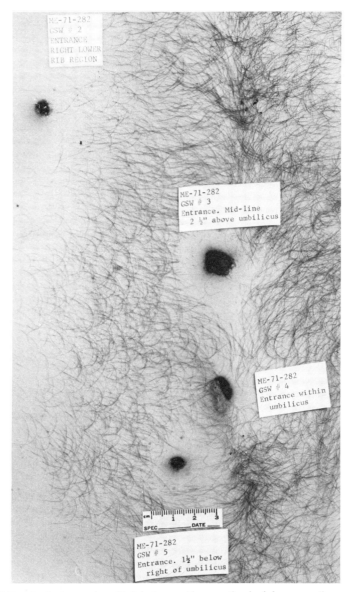

ME-71-282
GSW # 2
ENTRANCE
RIGHT LOWER
RIB REGION

ME-71-282
GSW # 3
Entrance. Mid-line
2 ½" above umbilicus

ME-71-282
GSW # 4
Entrance within
umbilicus

SPEC____ ____DATE____

ME-71-282
GSW # 5
Entrance. 1½" below
right of umbilicus

Fig. 10-3.   A photograph with labels: another method of documenting gunshot wounds.

and its distance from the top of the head and from the midline. The chart will also provide, at a glance, information about the presence or absence of the effects of flame, smoke and gunpowder as well as the direction of the bullet through the body. Notes about the caliber of the

GUNSHOT WOUND INFORMATION CHART

Name of decedent: ___Ringo R. Rinker___

City or County: Broward County

		WOUND NO.							
		1		2		3		4	
		Ent.	Ex.	Ent.	Ex.	Ent.	Ex.	Ent.	Ex.
1. Location of Wound:	Head								
	Neck								
	Chest	x							
	Abdomen								
	Back								
	Arm Right								
	Arm Left								
	Leg Right								
	Leg Left								
2. Size of Wound:	Diam.	1/3"							
	Width								
	Length								
3. Inches from Wound to:	Top of Head	16"							
	Right of Midline								
	Left of Midline	3"							
4. Flame, Smoke and Gunpowder Effects:	On Skin	x							
	Clothing								
	Absent								
5. Direction of Bullet Through Body:	Backward	x							
	Forward								
	Downward								
	Upward	20°							
	To Right	40°							
	To Left								
6. Bullet Found:	Caliber	x							
	Shotgun								

Photographs made: Yes _x_ No____   X-rays made: Yes _x_ No____

REMARKS: The bullet entered the skin and subcutaneous tissues on the front of the left side of the chest. It entered the chest cavity between the 4th and 5th left ribs in the midclavicular line, passed backwards, 20° upwards and 40° to the right. It perforated the anterior margin of the upper lobe of the left lung, the ascending aorta and the upper lobe of the right lung. It exited from the chest between the 2nd and 3rd right ribs in the posterior axillary line. The bullet was found lodged under the skin of the back 5" from the midline and 14" from the top of the head. It weighed 92 grains and its base measured 3/8" in diameter.

Examined by: ___*Jerry J. Joshua*___   Date: ___January 1, 1975___
Jerry J. Joshua, M. D.

Fig. 10-4.   Gunshot wound information chart; hypothetical data filled in.

bullet and whether or not photographs and x-rays were made will also be reflected. In the space provided for "Remarks" the examiner should describe the course of the bullet from the point of entry to the exit, indicating the tissues and the organs perforated, and give the angles of the bullet track with the horizontal and vertical planes. If the bullet is recovered from the body, the exact location of lodgement in the body should be described. The condition of the bullet can be described in short by using the words "deformed," "flattened" or "intact." The bullet should be weighed, and if its base is not deformed, the diameter of the base should be measured. These measures should be recorded. Hypothetical data is filled in in the accompanying chart (Fig. 10-4) to serve as an example.

If an exit wound can be associated with an entrance wound, such an exit wound should be documented on the Gunshot Wound Information Chart in the column next to the column carrying information about the entrance wound. If an exit wound cannot be positively associated with a certain entrance wound, this should be stated in the space provided for remarks.

The wound numbering system should be consistent. The photographs, body diagrams and the gunshot wound information chart should all reflect the same number for a certain wound. Such an approach not only makes documentation easy, but also presentation of evidence in court from such records at a later date becomes convenient.

Once the body diagrams are properly completed and the gunshot wound information chart filled, all necessary information is documented. Detailed descriptions are then not necessary.

INTERNAL EXAMINATION

Principal objectives of internal examination in a case of a gunshot wound are retrieval of the missile (or pellets and wads), identification of the bullet track and determination of direction of fire, evaluation of internal injuries caused by the bullet, assessment of the role of disease, if any, and collection of articles of evidence.

The body may be opened with a primary Y-shaped incision. After the body is opened and the track of the bullet identified, the direction of fire should be recorded by noting the angles with the horizontal and vertical planes the bullet track makes from the point of entry. If the bullet strikes a bone and changes its course, the direction of fire may be evaluated with reference to the point of impact with the bone. If the bullet enters a hollow viscus or enters the blood stream, it may not be found at the end of the bullet track.

When the bullet is localized in the tissues, it should be carefully removed. A bullet may be squeezed out of the area of its lodgement with fingers after cutting the tissues around it. Clamps or forceps should not be used to extract the bullet, for they may disturb important markings on the bullet. If the bullet is lodged within a bone, such as a vertebra, after precisely localizing the bullet the bone should be sawn a short distance away from the bullet. After the bone with the bullet in it is excised, further breaking up of the excised piece of bone will help dislodge the bullet without damaging it. Every effort should be made to retrieve any fragments of bullet in the body also. A considerable

REPORT OF AUTOPSY

DECEDENT ___Ringo___ R. ___Rinker___ Autopsy authorized by: Kenneth K. King, M.D., M.E.
First name   Middle name   Last name   Name   Official Title

TYPE OF DEATH:	Unattended by a physician ☐	RIGOR		LIVOR		Body Identified by:
Violent or Unnatural ☒	Sudden in apparent health ☐	JAW ☒ ARMS ☐		COLOR Purple		Body tag on
Means: Gun	Unusual ☐ In prison ☐	NECK ☐ CHEST ☐		ANTERIOR POSTERIOR ☒		left big toe
	Suspicious ☐	BACK ☐ ABDOMEN ☐		LATERAL ☐		PERSONS PRESENT AT AUTOPSY
		LEGS ☐		REGIONAL		

AGE 25 RACE Negro SEX Male LENGTH 72" WEIGHT 170 lb EYES Brown PUPILS: R 6 mm. OPACITIES, ETC. Kenneth K. King,
HAIR Black BEARD -- MUSTACHE Black CIRCUMCISED Yes BODY HEAT Cool L 6 mm. M.D.

NON FATAL WOUNDS, SCARS, TATTOOING, OTHER FEATURES: Warm in flexures

An abrasion, 1 1/2 x 1", center of forehead.
See attached protocol, gunshot wound chart and x-rays.

PATHOLOGICAL DIAGNOSIS

1. Gunshot wound of chest:
   Perforation of fifth left rib anteriorly, perforation of anterior and posterior walls
   of left ventricle and pericardium 2" from apex.

2. Bilateral hemothorax: 1,000 c.c. blood left side, 200 c.c. right side.

3. Hemopericardium: 50 c.c.

4. Abrasion, forehead.

5. Adenoma, left adrenal.

Comment: A 0.22 calibre bullet lodged in subcutaneous tissues of back at the level of 9th
interspace, 4" to the left of midline, was retrieved and retained.

Probable cause of death:
Gunshot wound of chest.

PROVISIONAL REPORT ☐
FINAL REPORT ☒

A true copy: The facts stated herein are true and correct to the best
                                            of my knowledge and belief.
                                            Jerry J. Joshua, M.D.
                     1-1-73   Signature of Pathologist   City Hospital
_____   10 a.m. to 1 p.m. 1/1/73   Durham, N.C.
Chief Medical Examiner   Date   Date and time of autopsy   Place of autopsy

Fig. 10-5. A facsimile of the front page of the autopsy report recommended for
medicolegal cases; hypothetical data filled in.

amount of patience may be required to retrieve a missile from the body.
The bullet often is one of the most valuable pieces of evidence in a case
of homicidal shooting, hence no efforts must be spared to retrieve it. If
necessary, repeated x-rays should be made to localize and find the
bullet.

After the bullet is retrieved, its weight and the diameter of its base
should be noted. It should then be placed in a cardboard container or
envelope, which should be sealed and signed by the pathologist. The
container should be identified with the name of the decedent, case

number, area from which the bullet was removed and the date of autopsy. Separate containers must be used for each bullet. Metal containers should be avoided. They may damage the bullet or destroy markings on it.

In every case, the internal examination must be complete. For instance, the examination of the brain, neck organs, genital organs, etc., should not be omitted even if the bullet injury is limited to some other area.

Internal injuries should be accurately documented, and sections of internal organs should be retained for microscopic examination. It is a good practice to obtain a blood sample from every case. Blood can be easily drawn with a syringe from the right ventricle, pulmonary trunk or aorta. It may be required for toxicological analyses and to determine the victim's blood group.

After the external and internal wounds are documented by description, diagrams and photographs, the dermal gunshot wounds should be excised and retained for microscopic and other examinations.

AUTOPSY PROTOCOL

The findings of the autopsy should be recorded at the time of examination of the body. The observations may be dictated or written down by the pathologist.

The autopsy report should include the details of identification of the body; date, time and place of examination; findings of external and internal examinations and the cause of death. A facsimile of the front page of the autopsy report, originated in Virginia and now used in many states, is shown in Figure 10-5. Such a format is recommended since it gives vital information at a glance. Details of the results of the external and internal examinations, x-rays, histological and toxicological studies, and opinions can be appended when a complete report is requested by any party. The completed report should be sent to the person authorizing the autopsy and to the proper authorities.

REFERENCES

1. Cowan, M. E. and Purdon, P. L.: A study of the "paraffin test". J. For. Sci., 12:19, 1967.
2. Krishnan, S. S. and Nichol, R. C.: Identification of bullet holes by neutron activation analysis and auto radiography. J. For. Sci., 13:519, 1968.

11

Homicide, Suicide or Accident?

In Chapter 8 many of the questions that arise in the course of investigation of a gunshot wound fatality are discussed. Questions about the range of fire, direction of fire, type of weapon, location of wounds, number of wounds and the cause of death have important bearing on the ultimate question of whether the death is a homicide, suicide or an accident. In a medicolegal investigation of a firearm fatality the most important issue without doubt is that of *manner* of death.

In most instances the circumstances of death and the findings of the investigation leave no doubt about the manner of death. However, in some cases the answers to many of the questions, including the question pertaining to the manner of death, are not obvious. In such cases all available information such as the findings of the scene investigation, autopsy and police investigation must be supplemented by ancillary investigations before the manner of death is classified.

In this chapter an epidemiologic survey of firearm deaths is presented, and specific aspects of homicidal, suicidal and accidental gunshot wounds are discussed.

EPIDEMIOLOGY

Knowledge of the epidemiologic pattern of gun-related deaths can be useful to the investigator. In view of the high incidence of firearm deaths in the United States, it is possible to study a large series of cases in order to gain some idea about the pattern of homicidal, suicidal and accidental shootings.

In a 1974 study, Fatteh and Hayes analysed data on 2087 firearm fatalities that occurred in 1970 and 1971 in North Carolina.[4] The findings with reference to age, sex, race and the manner of death are summarized below with a view to present information from a typical representative United States jurisdiction.

Table 11-1. Racial Distribution of Firearm Fatalities
with Reference to the Manner of Death
(North Carolina, 1970 and 1971)

	Homicide	Suicide	Accident	Undetermined Manner of Death
Caucasians	373	768	112	48
Negroes	605	71	47	26
Indians	28	5	3	1

Age, Sex, and Race

Of the total number of firearms victims (2,087), 1,727 were males and 360 females. According to the 1970 census there were 2.48 million males and 2.59 million females in the State of North Carolina; 1,301 of the firearms victims were Caucasians, 749 Negroes, and 37 Indians. Racial distribution of the cases with respect to the manner of death is presented in Table 11-1. The proportion of Negroes in the population of North Carolina in 1970 was 22 per cent.[9] The distribution of 2,012 cases with respect to the age of the victim is shown in Table 11-2. The distribution clearly indicates that a large majority of the victims were in the prime of life. The rate of firearm deaths during the years 1970 and 1971 in the whole state of North Carolina, based on preliminary population figures of the 1970 census, was found to be 20.57 per 100,000 persons.

Table 11-2. Firearm Fatalities in North Carolina
(1970 and 1971) by Age.*

Age (Years)	Homicides	Suicides	Accidents	Total
0-10	5	0	22	27
11-20	101	47	48	196
21-30	335	128	32	495
31-40	223	123	21	367
41-50	165	186	18	369
51-60	102	194	12	308
61-70	46	106	3	155
71+	15	60	3	78
Unknown	14	—	3	17
Total	1,006	844	162	2,012

*Cases with "undetermined" manner of death are not included.

Manner of Death

The investigative reports and death certificates provided information regarding the manner of death in each case. This was classified as homicide, suicide or accident; in cases in which the circumstances were not clear enough to allow a definite classification, the manner of death was labeled "undetermined." In the series there were 1,006 homicides, 844 suicides, 162 accidental deaths, and 75 "undetermined" cases (57 males and 18 females; 48 Caucasians, 26 Negroes, and 1 Indian). No other relevant information was available on these cases. For the purpose of simplification, further analysis of the data was carried out with reference to the manner of death only (i.e., suicide, homicide, and accident).

Suicides. There were 1,146 suicides from all causes in North Carolina during the 2 years 1970 and 1971. Of these, 844 were committed with guns; males outnumbered females by 696 to 148; and there were 768 Caucasians (633 males, 135 females), 71 Negroes (58 males, 13 females), and 5 Indians (all 5 males). The distribution of these cases in different age groups is presented in Table 11-2.

There was a fairly uniform spread of suicides over the 12 months of the year, with a slight increase in the spring and fall months, and a low figure for January. Also, there was uniform spread of suicides over the days of the week. The greatest number of suicides were committed during the hours between 8:00 AM and 4:00 PM; 62 per cent of the suicides were committed during the day (8:00 AM to 8:00 PM). Suicides were relatively uncommon during the middle of the night.

The geographic location of shooting could be determined in 590 cases. Of this group, a total of 528 suicidal shootings occurred in homes—487 inside the house and 41 outside. Suicides in open spaces and public areas were rare.

The anatomic location of fatal wounds was determined in 614 cases. The general area of the head including the face and the neck was the most common site, accounting for 417 cases. In 204 of these the fatal wound was in the right temple, in 58 the mouth, in 43 the forehead, in 15 the left temple, and in the remaining cases the general area of the head was designated but the exact location was not specified. There were 170 cases with the fatal gunshot wound in the left anterior region of the chest and 26 cases with fatal injury in the epigastric region. One victim shot himself in the right femoral region.

In this series of 844 suicides, 831 cases showed only one gunshot wound; in the remaining 13 cases two shots were fired. In 8 of these 13 each victim fired two shots in the chest; two victims had both gunshot wounds in the temple area and three victims had gunshot wounds in the head and the chest areas. The autopsy in each case showed that one of the two bullets had caused nonfatal injuries.

With regard to weapons used to commit suicides, information was available in the reports of only 574 cases. Of these 574, a pistol or a rifle was used in 433 cases; in 244 of these, the weapon was known to be a pistol, in 81 a rifle, and in 108 a "pistol or rifle." The 22-caliber pistol was the most common weapon. Shotguns were used in 141 instances, the most commonly used gauge was 12.

The data were analyzed to determine the percentage of suicides in which alcohol was a possible factor. In 153 of the 451 cases an analysis for alcohol was not done. From the results of analyses in 298 cases it was learned that the blood alcohol was negative in 60 per cent of the cases, and in those with positive results the average blood alcohol was 185 mg per 100ml (0.185%).

Homicides.   There were 1,292 homicides in North Carolina during 1970 and 1971; those committed by firearms numbered 1,006. Of the homicide victims 839 (83.4%) were males and 167 were females. A study of the racial distribution revealed a reversal of the suicide figures. Of all the murder victims 605 were Negroes, 373 Caucasians, and 28 Indians. The death toll included 502 Negro males accounting for almost 50 per cent of all homicides by guns. The highest number of murder victims (335) fell in the age group 21 to 30 years; the age group 31 to 40 years was the next highest with 223 fatalities (see table 11-2).

There was no clear-cut seasonal variation in the number of homicides. Perhaps just incidentally, the month of December showed the highest number. The information derived from the study of 761 homicides, however, clearly showed that a large proportion (386 of 761) occurred on Saturdays and Sundays. When the time of day was taken into consideration, it was found that 374 of the 761 victims were killed between 8:00 PM and 4:00 AM.

From the investigative reports it was possible to determine the location of homicidal shootings in 666 cases. Of this total, 355 were committed inside houses, 40 outside the homes, 91 on or near streets or roads, and 85 at nightspots such as bars, nightclubs, poolrooms, and cafés. Twenty persons were killed in automobiles, 14 at service stations, 19 at the decedent's place of work, and the remaining at miscellaneous places, which ironically included a church and a cemetery.

The anatomic sites of fatal wounds in 741 cases were also determined. In 383 cases the fatal wound was in the chest (front and back), in 179 the head and the neck, in 123 the abdomen, in 13 the extremities, and in 3 the buttocks. In 40 cases the wounds were inflicted at more than one of the above sites. It was possible to determine the number of shots fired in 756 cases: single shots were fired and proved fatal in 575 cases, two shots in 64 cases, three in 41, four in 25, five or more in 19, and "multiple" shots in 32 cases.

Analysis of the data in an attempt to determine the circumstances of fatal shooting was only partially fruitful: in only 339 cases could the cause of shooting and the activity of the victim be determined. In 229 cases the victim was involved in an argument or altercation; 34 persons were shot by robbers while defending themselves or their property; 19 were fatally wounded while they were attacking or threatening the assailant; 5 policemen were shot in the line of duty; and the remaining 26 persons were killed under other miscellaneous circumstances.

While ascertaining the circumstances of the shootings, the data regarding the identity of the persons committing the homicides were analyzed. The information on this aspect was available in 358 cases. In 162 instances the person doing the shooting was a member of the immediate family and in 111 a "friend."

Of the 704 cases in which the type of weapon could be ascertained, a shotgun was known to have been used in 164 cases, a pistol in 199, a rifle in 63, and a "pistol or rifle" in 278. The analysis revealed that .22 caliber pistols, .22 caliber rifles, and 12-gauge shotguns were the most commonly used weapons.

To evaluate the role of alcohol in the incidence of homicidal shootings, the available data on this aspect were analyzed. In only 464 cases were the analyses for alcohol in the blood of the victims requested and performed. The blood of 315 (68%) victims was found to contain alcohol. The average blood alcohol level in all cases with positive results was 202 mg per 100 ml (0.202%).

Accidents.   During the years 1970 and 1971 there were 162 deaths caused by accidental shootings. Of the victims 135 were males and the remaining 27 females. There were 112 Caucasians, 47 Negroes, and 3 Indians. The highest number of deaths occurred in the 11- to 20-year age group. Approximately 55 per cent of all accidental deaths from gunshot wounds occurred during the months October through February—months which make up the hunting season. There were more deaths on Saturdays than on any other day of the week, the largest number occurring between 4:00 PM and 8:00 PM. Among the 77 cases in which the information about the weapon was available, 30 deaths were caused by pistols, 20 by rifles, 9 by "pistols or rifles," and 18 by shotguns.

National Figures

An attempt has been made to compare the figures of firearm fatalities in different states. At the time of writing the latest figures available for the purpose of such comparison were for the year 1970. The figures for that year are presented in Table 11-3.[10] It is interesting that the southern states show a higher rate than the northern and the western states.

(Text continued on p. 147)

Table 11-3.   Firearm Fatalities in 1970 Classified by State

State	1970 Population in Millions (Bureau of Census)	Accidents Caused by Firearms	Suicides by Firearms and Explosives	Homicides Caused by Firearms and Explosives	Total Firearm Deaths*
United States	203.235	2406	11772	11213	25391 (12.5)
Alabama	3.444	111	236	311	658 (19.1)
Alaska	0.302	14	31	17	62 (20.5)
Arizona	1.772	44	178	94	316 (17.8)
Arkansas	1.923	45	154	150	349 (18.1)
California	19.953	179	1320	761	2260 (11.3)
Colorado	2.207	28	211	90	329 (14.9)
Connecticut	3.032	14	108	66	188 (6.2)
Delaware	0.548	1	28	25	54 (9.9)
District of Columbia	0.756	14	23	135	172 (22.8)
Florida	6.789	107	550	689	1346 (19.8)
Georgia	4.589	126	416	666	1208 (26.3)
Hawaii	0.769	4	20	21	45 (5.9)
Idaho	0.713	20	68	21	109 (15.3)
Illinois	11.113	116	422	739	1277 (11.5)
Indiana	5.193	56	289	201	546 (10.5)
Iowa	2.825	17	153	30	200 (7.1)
Kansas	2.249	26	164	76	266 (11.8)
Kentucky	3.219	39	264	252	555 (17.2)
Louisiana	3.643	89	251	347	687 (18.9)
Maine	0.993	7	73	10	90 (9.1)
Maryland	3.922	27	197	236	460 (11.7)
Massachusetts	5.689	20	116	95	231 (4.1)
Michigan	8.875	79	465	628	1172 (13.2)
Minnesota	3.805	28	169	56	253 (6.7)

*The numbers in parentheses represent the rate of deaths per 100,000 population. Cases with "undetermined" manner of death are not included.

(Table continued, overleaf)

Table 11-3.   Firearm Fatalities in 1970 Classified by State
(Continued)

State	1970 Population in Millions (Bureau of Census)	Accidents Caused by Firearms	Suicides by Firearms and Explosives	Homicides caused by Firearms and Explosives	Total Firearm Deaths*
Mississippi	2.216	57	126	234	417 (18.8)
Missouri	4.677	69	301	374	744 (15.9)
Montana	0.694	15	53	14	82 (11.8)
Nebraska	1.483	25	93	30	148 (10.0)
Nevada	0.488	6	77	31	114 (23.4)
New Hampshire	0.737	6	47	9	62 (8.4)
New Jersey	7.168	28	144	212	384 (5.4)
New Mexico	1.016	29	106	54	189 (18.6)
New York	18.241	48	388	775	1211 (6.6)
North Carolina	5.082	85	400	455	940 (18.5)
North Dakota	0.617	9	45	3	57 (9.2)
Ohio	10.652	77	602	532	1211 (11.4)
Oklahoma	2.559	63	178	116	357 (14.0)
Oregon	2.091	20	169	54	243 (11.6)
Pennsylvania	11.793	70	528	340	938 (8.0)
Rhode Island	0.949	1	20	14	35 (3.7)
South Carolina	2.590	51	222	324	597 (23.1)
South Dakota	0.666	16	29	6	51 (7.7)
Tennessee	3.924	74	370	327	771 (19.7)
Texas	11.196	201	870	1046	2117 (18.9)
Utah	1.059	19	83	21	123 (11.6)
Vermont	0.444	6	29	4	39 (8.8)
Virginia	4.648	57	352	303	712 (15.3)
Washington	3.409	25	250	75	350 (10.3)

Table 11-3. Firearm Fatalities in 1970 Classified by State (Continued)

State	1970 Population in Millions (Bureau of Census)	Accidents Caused by Firearms	Suicides by Firearms and Explosives	Homicides Caused by Firearms and Explosives	Total Firearm Deaths*
West Virginia	1.744	33	133	67	233 (13.4)
Wisconsin	4.417	49	209	65	323 (7.3)
Wyoming	0.332	11	42	6	59 (17.8)

*The numbers in parentheses represent the rate of deaths per 100,000 population. Cases with "undetermined" manner of death are not included.

HOMICIDAL GUNSHOT WOUNDS

The Medical Examiner or the Coroner, with the help of police, has initial responsibility for ruling on the manner of death so that proper charges may be filed in the cases of homicidal shooting. The medicolegal officers, in some jurisdictions, have access to most of the circumstantial and physical evidence and they are required to rule on the cause and manner of death. This is a serious task, and every aspect of the case must be carefully studied before a decision on the manner of death is rendered. When homicide is a possibility the following aspects of the case should be considered.

Circumstances of Shooting

In the majority of cases the circumstances of shooting are obvious from the accounts of the witnesses. Often simple arguments among relatives or friends result in shooting deaths, or altercations lead to fatal shooting. Some fatalities result from robbery attempts, and occasionally an innocent third party gets killed in the shooting spree or a police officer loses his life while enforcing law. Murder-suicide situations are usually self-explanatory. It is the unwitnessed murder that is not associated with any helpful circumstantial details that demands the most careful investigation to establish the manner of death.

The Scene of Death

In cases where reliable witnesses are not present at the scene of shooting, the investigator may find evidence suggestive of homicide. If burglary or robbery is the motive for murder, there may be evidence of

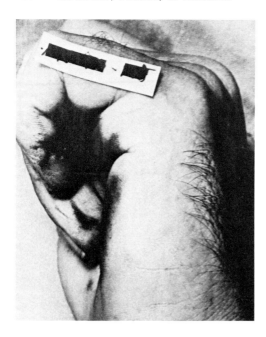

Fig. 11-1. A gunshot wound and gunpowder soiling on the hand.

ransacking. Struggle between the victim and the assailant may result in disarray of articles. The absence, at the scene of death, of the gun responsible for the fatality often gives a strong indication of homicide. The position of the victim may give a clue as to the manner of death. If an attempt has been made to move the body, the location of livor and the posture of the body might suggest involvement of another person in the death.

One of the possibilities that should always be kept in mind is that of alteration of the scene. The assailant may attempt to conceal the crime by making the scene look like a suicide or an accident. The weapon may be planted in the victim's hand or placed in a position suggestive of accident or suicide.

Examination of the Clothes and the Hands

In addition to the examination of gunshot wounds, the general examination of the body should be directed at the examination of the clothing and of the victim's hands. The presence of shot soiling around the bullet holes in the clothing may contribute to the determination of range of fire. The presence of only grease marks in the margins of the bullet hole, indicating long range fire, will suggest homicide or accident.

The dorsal aspects of the victim's hands may show the presence of

Fig. 11-2. A homicidal contact gunshot wound on the face.

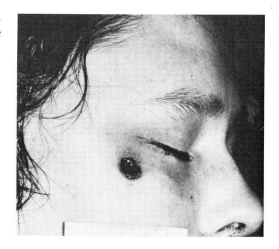

gunpowder or bullet wounds. Powder residue or grease may also be found on the palm of the victim's hand. If a homicide victim tries to ward off the attack, he may hold the muzzle of the gun. The shot fired in such circumstances would cause shot soiling on the victim's hand, and there may also be a gunshot wound on the hand (Fig. 11-1).

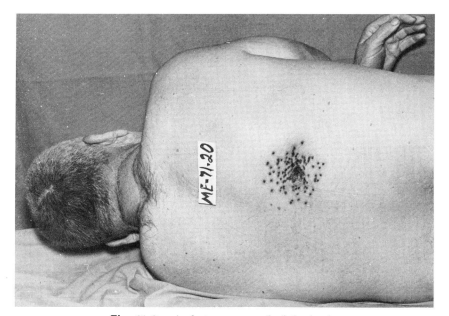

Fig. 11-3. A shotgun wound of the back.

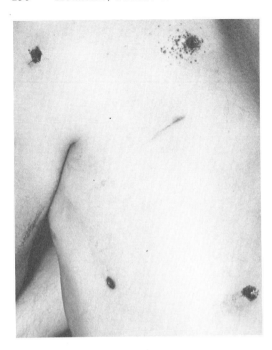

Fig. 11-4. Multiple homicidal gunshot wounds inflicted from different distances.

Examination of Wounds

Location of Homicidal Wounds on the Body. These wounds can be seen on any part of the body. Wounds on the face (Fig. 11-2), on the back (Fig. 11-3) and on a body part inaccessible for self-infliction, and multiple wounds (Fig. 11-4) should be presumed to be homicidal until accidental or suicidal infliction can be ruled out.

Homicidal wounds that are inflicted at the so called "classical" suicidal sites (see below) can create serious confusion especially if the circumstances of shooting are unclear. In the recent past this author has seen two cases of homicidal contact gunshot wounds of the center of forehead. In one instance, a burglar was supposed to have shot the victim in the center of the forehead with a bird shot (Fig. 11-5). The victim also had a contact gunshot wound at the back of the head. In another instance, a 31-year-old Negro male shot by an unknown assailant was found dead lying on the street. He was shot in the center of the forehead with a 0.38 caliber gun. The wound was a contact one with flame, smoke and gunpowder effect. On rare occasions, homicide victims show contact gunshot wounds in the temple region, in the neck (Fig. 11-6) and in the heart area. Such cases should be interpreted with care. The following unusual case was investigated by G. T. Mann, M.D.

Fig. 11-5. A homicidal contact gunshot wound in the center of the forehead inflicted with No. 12 bird shot.

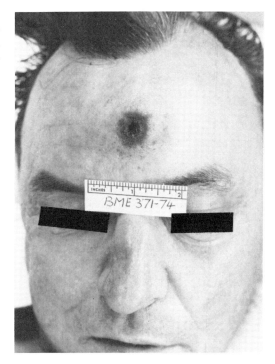

An autopsy on a woman revealed two gunshot wounds—one in the chest and the other in the right temple region. The pathologist noted marked differences in the features of the two wounds. The one in the chest had features indicating that it was inflicted before death. The other wound in the temple region was devoid of any hemorrhage in the skin and subcutaneous tissues and there was no hemorrhage in the brain indicating that this was inflicted after death. The information relayed to the assailant through police led to confession. The assailant admitted that he had shot the victim in the chest and then to make it appear suicide he had shot her in the temple region after she was dead.

Homicidal shooting through the mouth is rare. According to Polson it is "likely only when the victim is sleeping, drunk or drugged." However, he goes on to describe a case in which a girl asked her boy friend to close his eyes and open his mouth, and when he did so she fired a shot into his mouth.[6] Fatteh has described a case in which a woman was teasing her husband by putting her tongue out.[2] The husband stuck the muzzle of a 0.22 caliber rifle in her mouth and shot her. He tendered a plea to second degree murder and was sentenced to thirty years imprisonment. Necropsy showed a contact entrance wound near the tip of the tongue (Fig. 11-7). The bullet exited from the dorsal aspect of the tongue near the pharynx. It travelled backward and left the body at the top part

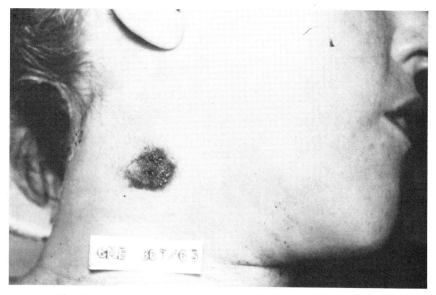

Fig. 11-6.   A homicidal contact gunshot wound of the neck.

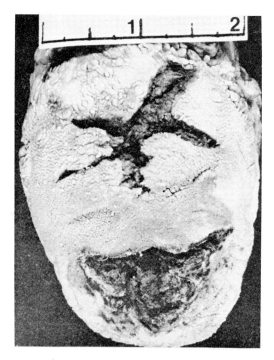

Fig. 11-7. A homicidal contact gunshot wound of the tongue. The entrance wound is near the tip and the exit away from it. (Fatteh, A.: Homicidal gunshot wound of mouth. J. For. Sci. Soc., *12*:348, 1972.)

Fig. 11-8. A homicidal gunshot wound of the mouth.

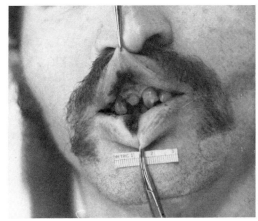

of the back of the neck. In another instance, a sheriff's deputy was shot in the mouth by a man who was being arrested. In a more recent case, a man shot his friend during an argument over a girlfriend. The bullet entered the mouth in the midline between the lips (Fig. 11-8). Both lips showed bullet grazes at the apposing points. The bullet perforated the tongue and entered the cranium through the posterior pharynx. Death resulted from severance of the medulla.

Since most of the gunshot wounds of the mouth are suicidal, a homicide with a gunshot wound in the mouth may be misinterpreted. In suicides, the victim points the muzzle upwards and the entrance wound is in the palate or posterior pharynx (Fig. 11-9). The tongue almost always escapes injury. If the bullet injures the tongue, the case should arouse strong suspicion that the shot was not a self-inflicted one (Fig. 11-10).

Wounds at multiple anatomic locations on the body must be considered homicidal until proved otherwise, even if they are contact or close-range wounds. In one case described by Gonzales et al., the perpetrator fired shots at close range in a straight line at equal intervals into the victim's right chest, flank, hip and thigh.[5]

Range of Fire. Homicidal gunshot wounds may be caused by contact, close-range or distant shots. A majority of homicidal wounds are inflicted from a range of more than an arm's reach. Such cases usually do not pose significant problems. However, wounds caused from contact or close-range shots have to be carefully evaluated to exclude the possibility of suicide or accident.

Direction of Fire. The consideration of gunshot wounds in relation to the bullet tracks, points of lodgement of the bullets in the body and the exit wounds helps to establish the direction of fire. The determina-

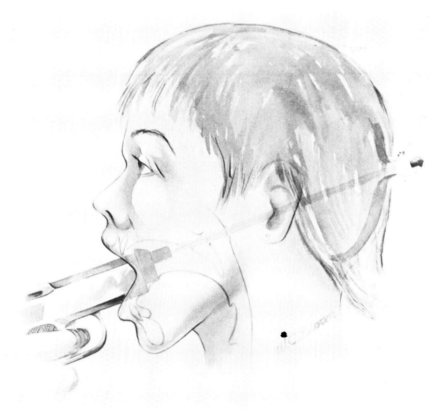

Fig. 11-9.   A diagram illustrating the features of suicidal gunshot wounds of the mouth. (Fatteh, A.: Homicidal gunshot wound of mouth. J. For. Sci. Soc. 12:374, 1972.)

tion of the direction of fire can help, in some cases, to establish that certain wounds are not self-inflicted.

Multiple Guns.   On rare occasions the victim may be fired at by more than one assailant or he may be caught in a cross-fire. In such situations there may be wounds on the body caused by more than one gun.

Disposal of the Body after Shooting

When a body is removed from the place of shooting (except for the possible purpose of treatment of injuries) or if an attempt is made to dispose of the body, commission of crime becomes obvious. The criminal may try to conceal the crime by dumping the body on the roadside away from the place of shooting, by throwing it in a river, canal or sea, or by burning it in a car, house or in a secluded spot. He may simply

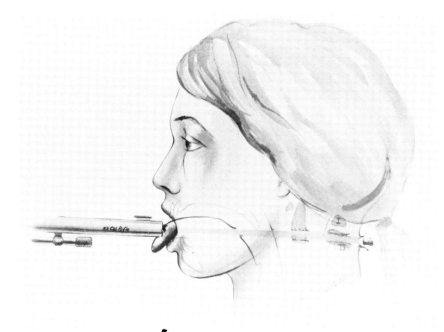

Fig. 11-10. A diagram illustrating the features of homicidal gunshot wounds of mouth. (Fatteh, A.: Homicidal gunshot wound of mouth. J. For. Sci. Soc., *12*:357, 1972.)

bury it in the ground. An attempt may be made to dispose of the body after dismembering it. Decomposition of the body, burning, dismemberment and other postmortem injuries may render the investigation difficult. However, a complete investigation would disclose the truth as illustrated by the following cases.

1. One day parts of the body of a man were found in a burned automobile. The automobile was a Pontiac with license plates that had been allocated to a Cadillac. In the car there were 24 bottles of "moonshine." The charred body consisted of the torso and several portions of bones. Except for a small portion of patterned underpants, all clothing was burned. With the body were a brass belt buckle with a name engraved on it, a wristwatch and a key ring with 12 keys. The head was missing with the level of separation at C2. This was also seen on x-rays which did not show any radioopaque objects in the body. There was some froth in the trachea and the main bronchi but no soot. The lungs were congested and edematous. No natural disease was found. There was some unburned, light brown hair in the pubic area. The decedent's blood type was B, blood alcohol level was 290 mg. per 100 ml. and the carboxyhemoglobin saturation was 15 per cent.

The following day, a head and the hand were found 3½ miles from where the charred body was found. The head and hand were buried in a 2-foot-deep hole on a farm (Fig. 11-11). Examination of the head showed a contact gunshot

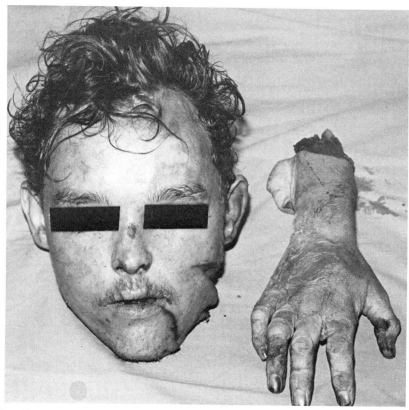

Fig. 11-11.   A shooting murder. The head and hand were removed before the rest of the body was burned in an automobile.

wound behind the left ear with an exit hole on the right side of the head. The head had been severed at the level of C2. The hair on the head and on the hand was light brown. Examination of the blood from the head showed alcohol concentration of 290 mg. per 100 ml., blood type B and negative carboxyhemoglobin.

The head was identified by visual identification of the face as being that of a 21-year-old man. The fingerprints from the hand and a scar on the wrist identified the hand as belonging to the same man. The circumstances and autopsy findings revealed several points that matched the charred remains with the head, leaving no doubt that all the remains were of one man. The personal effects found with the charred remains were identified as belonging to a man who was later convicted of the murder of this man. The convict had attempted to fake his own death in order to collect insurance in the amount of $250,000.00.

2. The body of a 45-year-old male was concealed in the corner of a large warehouse by pouring wet cement over it. The cement solidified in a neat block measuring approximately 6 × 3 × 3 feet. However, decomposition fluids started to pour out from the unsealed portions at the bottom of the cement block, causing a foul odor. This raised questions and complaints from the warehouse

workers. Out of fear of being caught, the assailant broke the cement block during one night, removed the body and transported it to another area about 135 miles from the warehouse. This was done about two weeks after the body was sealed in cement. At the new location the body was buried in ground. Telephone tips led the police to search that area. The assailant suspected that the police might discover the body, so he dug it up and reburied it in the ground not too far from where he dug it up. By this time widespread search of the area was underway. About 5 weeks after the cement block was broken for removal of the body, the remains were spotted by the police in a shallow grave.

The body had been wrapped in plastic sheets which were tied with strings. Large pieces of cement were found with the body and portions of plastic sheets and strings were embedded in the pieces of cement indicating that the body had probably been wrapped in plastic sheets before the wet cement was poured. Around the body and the sheets was a blanket and a large rug. The body was in an advanced state of decomposition. However, it was possible to obtain good fingerprints and the identification of the decedent was made from these.

At autopsy, entrance gunshot wounds were found in a 4-inch diameter area of the left upper chest between the nipple and the left shoulder. Three bullets were retrieved from under the skin in the right axillary line. The lungs and the arch of the aorta were perforated and four ribs fractured by bullets.

The gun alleged to have been used in the crime was discovered after a tip-off. It too had been concealed in cement poured around it. Ballistic work confirmed that the bullets found in the body had been fired by the gun retrieved from cement.

A close associate of the victim, who owned the warehouse and the property where the body was buried and reburied and who had access to the place where the gun was found, was charged with first degree murder and convicted.

SUICIDAL GUNSHOT WOUNDS

The investigation of suicides committed with firearms usually reveals a combination of facts that makes the manner of death clear. Some of the salient features that prove helpful in the investigation of a suicide are (1) the history of problems causing depression; (2) the presence of a suicide note; (3) the presence of the gun near the body; (4) election of a "classical" site on the body for infliction of the wound; and (5) the presence of a contact or close-range wound on the body. Suicides can present a wide variety of situations that can make the determination of the manner of death difficult. Commonly observed features of suicides and several unusual variations are discussed here to give an overall picture of suicidal gunshot wounds.

The Scene of Death

The person contemplating suicide usually selects a secluded place such as a closed room or wooded area to end his life. Hence, most of the suicides are unwitnessed. However, this is not always so. In a fit of depression a person may take his own life in the presence of another person. Examples of suicides by armed individuals who are being arrested are seen from time to time. An unusual suicide occurred in Florida recently: a young woman in charge of broadcasting a morning show on television placed the gun against her temple and fired the shot while she was on the air.

Personal History of the Victim

In any investigation of a possible suicide, the personal history of the victim must be thoroughly explored. The inquiries might reveal that the decedent had social, marital or economic problems. There may be history of depression from long-standing problems or sudden reverses and failures. Information about suicide threats and attempts may also be available. Consultation with the decedent's doctor may reveal previous psychiatric problems. Occasionally there is absolutely nothing in the personal history of the victim to indicate suicide even though every other piece of evidence points to such a verdict.

Suicide Note

A suicide note, if found, gives one of the best clues to the manner of death. However, only about a quarter of the victims leave suicide notes. The notes in most instances are handwritten but they may be typed, and rarely the suicide message may be taped. If the suicide note is handwritten, the handwriting should be checked to see if it resembles the victim's other writings. Most times the suicide note is in the vicinity of the victim's body. It may, however, be in another room of the house or relatives may hide it. In one case the victim had mailed the note, which was received one day after the body was found.

Position of the Gun Relative to the Body

The position of the gun in relation to the body can vary a great deal. In most of the cases of suicidal shooting the gun is near the body. If a handgun is used, it may still be in the hand that fired it. If it is in the hand, it will be held loosely unless cadaveric spasm caused it to be grasped tightly. Sometimes it is near the firing hand and occasionally it is several feet away from the body. The gun may bear the victim's fingerprints. There may be blood and hair inside or on the muzzle. If a long-barreled gun is used, the trigger, when accessible, may be pulled with a finger. If not, it may be pulled with a toe or an attached string or stick.

At times the gun is not found at the scene of shooting. If the shooting occurs at home, the relatives may have taken away the gun. In cases of suicides occurring outdoors, the gun may be stolen.

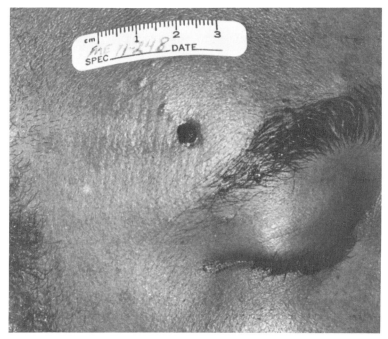

Fig. 11-12. A gunshot wound caused with a gun held tightly in contact with the skin (Fatteh, A.: Homicide or Suicide. J. For. Med., *122*:18, 1971).

A young man was found dead, slumped over the steering wheel of his car, which was parked in a parking lot. There was a contact gunshot wound in the right temple and a suicide note in the front shirt pocket. Also, there was gunpowder on his right hand. The gun, probably stolen, was never found.

In another case, a middle-aged man was found dead in the woods about 100 yards from the road. He had a contact gunshot wound in the right temple. Investigation revealed that he had been depressed and had told two of his friends that he was going to take his own life. His glasses, hat and shoes were found near the body. The gun was missing.

Examination of the Victim's Hands

The hand that fired the shot may show evidence of gunsmoke, gunpowder deposits and traces of metals. With the use of handguns, the effects of the components of a shot are seen commonly on the thumb, index finger and the area between them. Gunpowder, trace metal and smoke effect may be seen on both hands if the victim tries to stabilize the gun with two hands while shooting.

The hand firing the shot may also show a pattern of gun parts. For instance, one may see a pressure impression of the trigger on the ventral aspect of the index finger, impression of the trigger guard and that of the compensator may be seen.

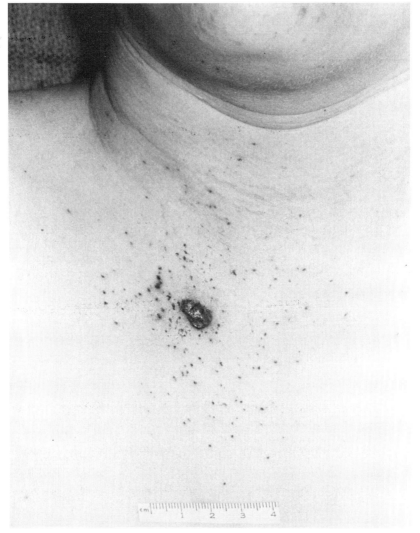

Fig. 11-13.   A suicidal gunshot wound inflicted from a muzzle–target distance of about 4 inches.

At the moment the shot is fired the hand pulling the trigger is close to the wound. Consequently, blood spatters soil the gun and the hand. In cases of suicide, therefore, blood spatters should be looked for on the hands.

The presence of old scars or recent incisions on the wrist will suggest a previous suicide attempt.

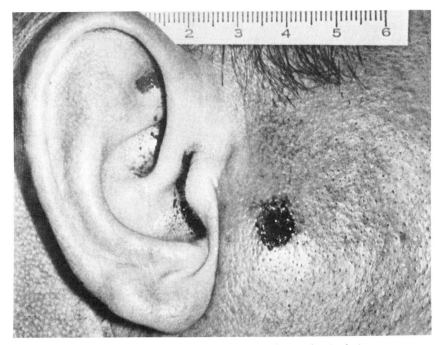

Fig. 11-14.   A suicidal gunshot wound at a classical site.

Range of Fire

Self-inflicted wounds are usually contact or close-range wounds. Therefore, the flame, smoke and gunpowder effects are seen in most cases. A gun held in tight contact with the skin might produce a wound that may lack such effects (Fig. 11-12). If the shot is fired in the precordial region or in the epigastrium, the victim may move the clothing away from the target area. When this is not done, the clothing will show distinct flame, smoke and gunpowder effects.

Only in rare instances is the shot not fired from contact range. A go-go dancer shot herself in the left upper chest region when her boyfriend threatened to leave her (Fig. 11-13). Test fires showed that the shot was fired from a distance of about 4 inches.

Direction of Fire

The direction of fire can be of help in the reconstruction of the events of suicidal shooting. The bullets fired in the temple region generally travel more or less toward the opposite temple, those in the mouth travel backwards and upwards, and the bullets entering the precordial region and the epigastrium ordinarily are directed in the backward

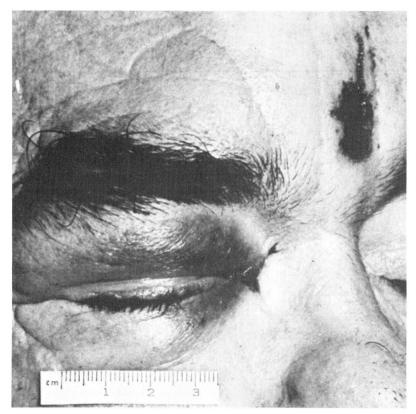

Fig. 11-15.   A suicidal gunshot wound in the center of the forehead.

direction. The investigator should try to evaluate the direction of fire with reference to the gun involved to see if the course of the bullet within the body is consistent with suicidal infliction of the wound. If the course indicates deviation from the general pattern, the possibility of accident or homicide should be considered.

Location of Suicidal Wounds on the Body

Suicide victims elect "classical" sites. Based on the results of a study of 844 suicides, the sites chosen to inflict suicidal gunshot wounds, in order of frequency, are the temple area (right temple by right-handed persons and left temple by left-handed persons), heart area, mouth and the center of the forehead.

Suicidal Gunshot Wounds of the Head.   A contact gunshot wound in the temple area (Fig. 11-14) or in the dead center of the forehead (Fig. 11-15) with blackening of the skin margins poses no difficulty in in-

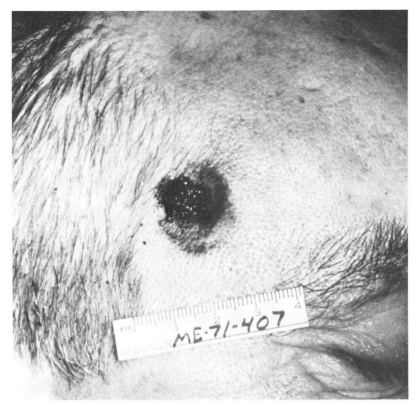

Fig. 11-16.   A contact suicidal gunshot wound of the temple.

terpretation, especially if supporting evidence in favor of suicide is available. The presence of such wounds, however, does not exclude the possibility of homicide (Fig. 11-5). Suicidal wounds are most commonly present in front of the upper half of the ear. Often they are located just above the ear (Fig. 11-16). Occasionally suicidal wounds are seen just behind the ear. With an entry wound behind the ear or in an area away from the classical suicidal site, however, the possibility of homicide should be excluded (Figs. 11-17, 11-18, 11-19).

Suicidal wounds may sometimes be found at unusual locations on the head. In the following instance a suicidal gunshot wound was found at a site most presumptive of homicide—the vertex of the head.

A young man who was known to dislike guns bought a 0.22 caliber rifle to shoot himself. He found privacy in an unused cottage garage. Suspending a rope from a beam, he attached the gun pointing downward. By placing the muzzle at the back of his head, he pulled the trigger by means of a curtain rod curved at one end, shooting himself. This man had marital and financial problems, he had been depressed, and he did leave a suicide note.

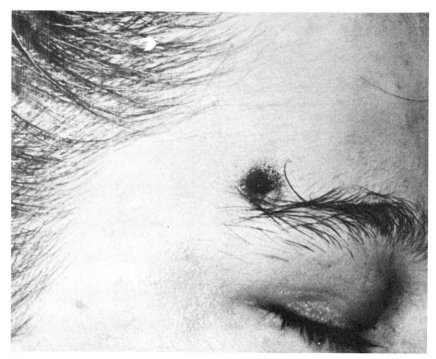

Fig. 11-17. A gunshot wound immediately above the eye. Such a wound should arouse suspicion of foul play.

Polson also has described a case of suicidal gunshot wound at the back of the head.[6] In that case a Portuguese student contrived to fire a shotgun to produce an entrance wound at the back of his head. The possibility of homicide was completely excluded by the police.

Gonzales et al. described a case in which the deceased had held the gun vertically downward on top of the head and shot himself.[5] These authors indicate that "in a few cases the suicide interposes his hand between the pistol and his head shooting himself through the palm of the hand" and also states that "some suicides insert the muzzle of the gun in the nares. . . . ".

The features of suicidal and homicidal gunshot wounds of the mouth have already been discussed.

An entrance wound on the face must arouse suspicion of foul play and in a case of a wound around the eye the possibility of a crime should be ruled out before a verdict of suicide or accident is rendered. Suicidal persons do not like to shoot through the eye. The study of the English literature did not reveal a single case of suicidal gunshot wound through the eye. This author had the opportunity of seeing an exceptional case recently. The facts of the case were as follows:

A 27-year-old left-handed male was found dead lying on a hotel room floor with a 0.22 caliber automatic between his feet. Examination of the body re-

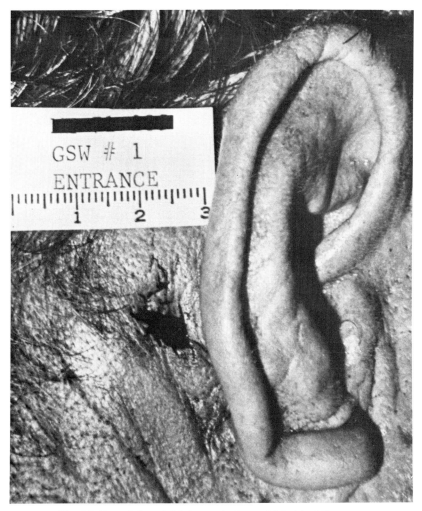

Fig. 11-18. A homicidal gunshot would behind the ear.

vealed a contact gunshot wound in the lower margin of the left upper eyelid (Fig. 11-20). The eyeball was perforated. The bullet travelling upwards, backwards and to the right was found lodged in the right parietal lobe of the brain. At the scene of death a suicide note was found. It read, "Have found it so hard and I find it so harder my world is closing in on me so I must take the easy way out." The handwriting on the note was confirmed to be the decedent's. The decedent had been depressed over his father's committing suicide and the family fighting over a five-million-dollar inheritance. The analysis of blood revealed the alcohol concentration of 100 mg per cent.

In another instance, a man arrested for an automobile violation shot himself in the eye in the presence of a witness.*

---

*Wiecking, D.K.: Personal communication, 1975.

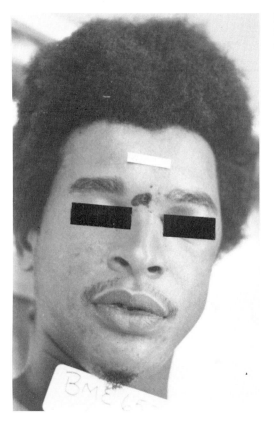

Fig. 11-19. A suicidal gunshot wound between the eyes.

Suicidal Gunshot Wounds of the Neck.   Suicidal gunshot wounds of the neck are uncommon. The neck is more apt to be selected as the site of suicidal shooting when a rifle or shotgun is the weapon. This is because it is easier to stabilize the muzzle under the jaw or the chin. Almost all of the suicidal gunshot wounds of the neck are located under the jaw or the chin. Wounds at any other location on the neck should arouse suspicion of foul play or accident.

Simpson has described an unusual case of gunshot wound of the back of the neck.[8] In that case the deceased had spent several weeks preparing an elaborate wooden frame to hold the rifle steady. Attached to the frame was a system of levers by which the rifle could be fired. The victim succeeded in firing a shot through the back of the neck.

Suicidal Gunshot Wounds of the Chest.   Most of these wounds are in the precordial region. Occasionally they may be slightly above or below the region of the heart. Suicidal gunshot wounds of the right side of the front of the chest are rare, as are the wounds of either side of the chest.

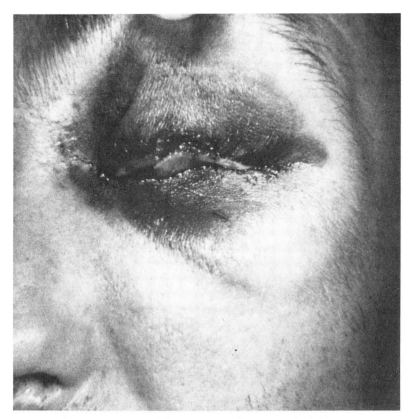

Fig. 11-20. Suicidal contact gunshot wound of the eye.

Suicidal Gunshot Wounds of the Abdomen.   These are most often inflicted in the epigastric region. Some place the muzzle under the rib cage. The weapon used is usually a rifle or a shotgun and the reason the epigastrium or the area under the rib cage is selected is that it is easier to stabilize the muzzle in that area. Gunshot wounds in other areas of the abdomen should be accepted as suicidal only if homicide and accident can be positively excluded. Six cases, each showing a gunshot wound in an area of the abdomen below the umbilicus, have been classified as suicides in one publication.[1] A mechanical arrangement set up to pull the trigger is often found at the scene in cases of suicide with gunshot wounds in the epigastrium and under the rib cage caused by long-barreled guns.

The missile tracks in cases of suicidal gunshot wounds of the abdomen are anterior to posterior.

Suicidal Gunshot Wounds of the Extremities.   These are extremely rare. One young man bled to death after he blasted the femoral vessels

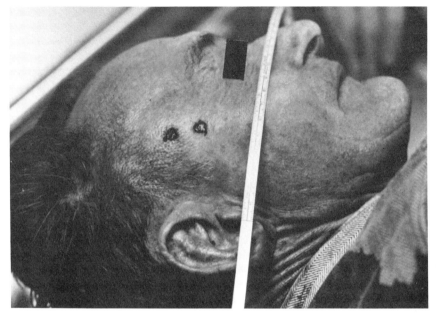

Fig. 11-21. Two suicidal gunshot wounds in the temple.

by placing the gun against the front of the right thigh. He pulled the trigger with the left great toe.

Multiple Suicidal Gunshot Wounds

Multiple suicidal gunshot wounds, though uncommon, do occur.[7] There may be two or more than two wounds. Thirteen cases, each with two gunshot wounds, have already been cited. An additional case with both gunshot wounds in the right temple area was investigated recently (Fig. 11-21). In most of the cases the circumstances of death are clear. Lack of circumstantial details can confuse the investigator. This author has reported a case with two suicidal gunshot wounds in the temple area (Fig. 11-22) in which only a complete investigation provided conclusive answers.[3] Discussion of cases with more than two suicidal gunshot wounds is presented in Chapter 13.

ACCIDENTAL GUNSHOT WOUNDS

Accidental shootings usually occur from defective guns. Children, hunters and intoxicated individuals are common victims. The sites of the wounds and the ranges vary a great deal. In a majority of the cases

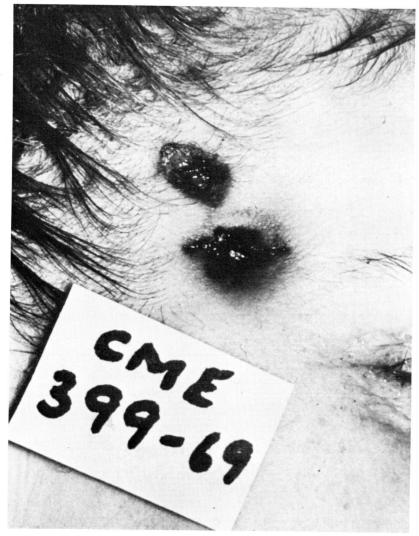

Fig. 11-22. Suicidal gunshot wounds in the temple. (Fatteh, A.: Homicide or Suicide. J. For. Med. *122*:18, 1971.)

the circumstances of death clarify the manner of death. However, when the circumstances are not clear, every detail of the case should be considered to rule out the possibility of suicide or homicide.

Russian roulette is a game in which the participants use a revolver loaded with one cartridge, the position of the loaded cylinder being unknown. Each player in turn places the muzzle of the revolver against his temple and pulls the trigger. If one happens to fire the only cartridge in the revolving drum, he gets killed. Such a death should be classified *accidental* since the participant does not intend to kill himself.

UNDETERMINED MANNER OF DEATH

By the time the scene investigation, the autopsy and the special investigative procedures are completed, the manner of death is clear in most cases. However, there may be an occasional case in which it is not possible to determine the manner of death. Such a problem may arise if there is total lack of circumstantial details or if the body is in an advanced state of decomposition. In situations when the Medical Examiner or the Coroner feels that everything that should be done has been done, he is completely justified in giving the manner of death as "undetermined."

Portions of this chapter are reproduced from Fatteh, A. and Hayes, W. C.: Firearm fatalities: epidemiologic and investigational considerations, pp. 45-68. In Wecht, Legal Medicine Annual 1974. Courtesy of Appleton-Century-Crofts, Publishing Division of Prentice-Hall, Inc., New York.

REFERENCES

1. Canfield, T. M.: Suicidal gunshot wounds of the abdomen. J. For. Sci., *14*:445, 1969.
2. Fatteh, A.: Homicidal gunshot wound of mouth. J. For. Sci. Soc., *12*:357, 1972.
3. ———: Murder or suicide? J. Forensic Med., *18*:122,1971.
4. Fatteh, A. and Hayes, W. C.: Firearm Fatalities: Epidemiologic and Investigational Considerations. *In* Wecht, C. H. (ed): Legal Medicine Annual 1974, Appleton-Century-Crofts, 1974.
5. Gonzales, T. A., Vance, M., Helpern, M., and Umberger, C. J.: Legal Medicine Pathology and Toxicology. New York, Appleton-Century-Crofts, 1954.
6. Polson, C. J.: The Essentials of Forensic Medicine. Springfield, Charles C Thomas, 1965.
7. Rentoul, E. and Smith, H.: Glaister's Medical Jurisprudence and Toxicology, ed. 13. Edinburgh, Churchill Livingstone, 1973.
8. Simpson, K.(ed.): Taylor's Principles and Practice of Medical Jurisprudence. ed. 12. London, J. & A. Churchill, 1965.
9. U.S. Department of Commerce Advance Report. 1970 census of population of North Carolina.
10. U.S. Department of Health, Education and Welfare, Public Health Service: Vital Statistics of the United States—General Mortality, 1970.

12

Artefacts in Cases of Gunshot Wounds

According to *Dorland's Illustrated Medical Dictionary,* an artefact is "any artificial product; any structure or feature that is not natural, but has been altered by processing. The term is used in histology and microscopy for a tissue that has been mechanically altered from its natural state."[2] For the purpose of discussion of cases of gunshot wounds, this definition has been modified: any change caused or a feature introduced in a body after death that is likely to lead to misinterpretation of medicolegally significant antemortem findings is considered to be an artefact. In other words, an artefact is a finding that is adventitious or physiologically unrelated to the natural state of the body or the tissues or the disease processes to which the body was subjected prior to death.

A general review of various artefacts introduced during the period between death and the autopsy and those introduced during the performance of autopsy has been presented by Fatteh.[3] Various artefacts, in cases of gunshot wounds, that can cause misinterpretation are discussed in this chapter.

RECOGNITION OF ARTEFACTS

A forensic pathologist must be able to recognize firearm wounds, distinguish entrance from exit wounds, and draw conclusions about the range and direction of fire. In most circumstances these present no undue difficulty. However, on occasions, artefacts add to the difficulties of interpretation. These artefacts may be caused by treatment of the victim, or by decomposition of the body, embalming techniques or even autopsy procedures.

Artefacts Caused During Treatment

When a victim of gunshot wounds is admitted to the hospital, the external injuries may be modified by therapeutic procedures. The

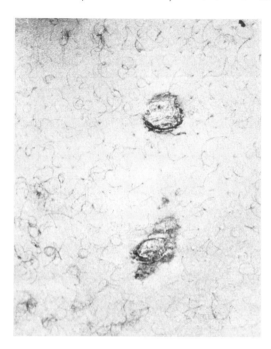

Fig. 12-1. Abdomen of a victim of three gunshot wounds showing two embalmer's trocar holes that were initially mistaken for gunshot wounds.

wounds may be scrubbed clean and medications may be applied. When this is done gunpowder or metallic fouling may be removed. Debridement of the wound will also result in the loss of these and other materials of evidential value. Excision of the wound margins and closure of the wound by sutures may make it difficult to identify correctly an entrance or an exit wound. During hospitalization the victim may "sustain" additional "pseudo-gunshot wounds." Drainage incisions in the chest and abdomen may also create problems. A complicated situation may be created by surgical extension of a gunshot wound. A classical example of this is what may be termed the Kennedy phenomenon: surgical alteration of the gunshot wound on the neck of President John F. Kennedy, the difficulty in the evaluation of that wound and the subsequent controversies about whether it was an entrance or an exit wound are well known.

Decomposition Artefacts

In decomposed bodies gunshot wounds are sometimes greatly modified. With the skin slippage there may be loss of hair and loss of gunpowder from the skin around an entrance wound. The margins of an entry wound may become ragged due to disintegration of the tissue at the margins. These effects may alter the wounds so much that it may be difficult to differentiate an entrance wound from an exit wound. The size and shape of a gunshot wound may also be considerably altered by decomposition. In one case of multiple gunshot wounds, a wound was twice the size of the others because intestinal loops had protruded through it.

Embalming Artefacts

In the United States, with rare exceptions, all bodies are embalmed before burial. The embalming may be arterial through incisions at the sites of approachable arteries or with a trocar introduced through the abdominal wall. The embalmer may enlarge a gunshot wound to approach an artery or he may introduce a trocar through a missile wound and modify its dimensions. In a case with multiple gunshot wounds, trocar holes may add to the difficulties (Fig. 12-1). Since the skin and the subcutaneous tissues are rendered bloodless and fixed by embalming, the gunshot wounds sustained during life may closely resemble trocar holes (Fig. 12-2). In addition, the trocar may disturb the track of the bullet within the body and may even create false tracks. Such false tracks may result in misinterpretation of direction and angle of fire. The external appearances of the wounds will be greatly altered in other ways by the embalming process. The gunpowder around an entrance wound may be washed or scrubbed away by the embalmer during the general cleaning of the body. The features of the wounds may be further altered by the stitching up of the wounds and the application of make-up.

Artefacts on X-Rays

In the autopsy room, the examination should begin with careful search of the clothing. There may be loose bullets, fired and unfired, in the clothing. Pockets should be examined for unspent ammunition. If there are any loose cartridges in the clothing and the body is x-rayed with the clothes on, such cartridges will create confusion. X-rays may also depict other metallic objects, such as buttons, which may resemble bullets. Sometimes pieces of rocks make shadows on x-rays resembling missile shadows. In order to avoid misinterpretation from these extraneous objects it is advisable to x-ray the body after it is undressed and all objects that are likely to produce confusing shadows are removed.

Even after such precautions, artefactual shadows may be seen in the x-rays of the body. In the cases of gunshot wounds of the head, for instance, fillings in the teeth or crowns of teeth may resemble bullets or pellets on x-rays. If a crown or a filling is displaced from its original position, the interpretation of the x-ray film may be rendered difficult (Fig. 12-3).

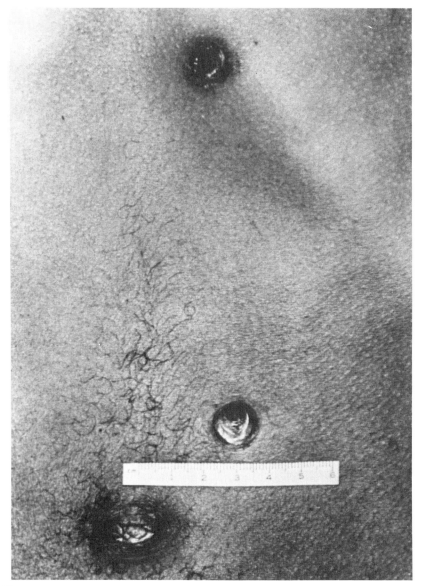

Fig. 12-2.   The lower hole is an embalmer's trocar hole, which resembles the gunshot wound above.

Burton has reported an interesting case of "missile" artefact.[1] His report concerns a 23-year-old man who "collapsed" at the wheel while driving a car. He sustained a head injury and became unconscious. On

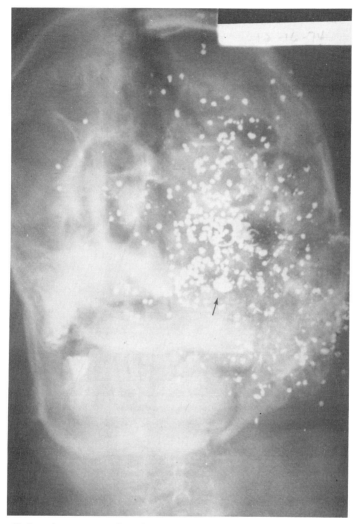

Fig. 12-3.   An x-ray with a displaced tooth crown resembling a bullet.

admission to the hospital he was in deep coma with profound shock. A stellate laceration at the vertex of the skull and a puncture wound in the left shoulder region were noted. X-rays of the chest revealed hemothorax and a metallic foreign body anterior to the body of the fourth thoracic vertebra. A clinicial diagnosis of gunshot wound of the chest with the entrance wound in the left shoulder was made. Repeat x-rays after 48 hours indicated migration of the metallic foreign body from the chest to the upper quadrant of the abdomen. Esophagoscopy

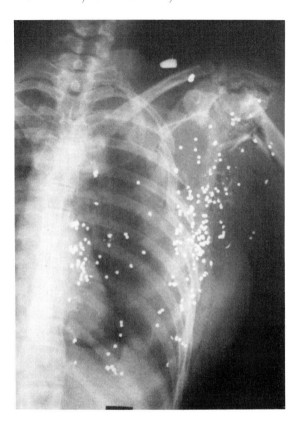

Fig. 12-4. An x-ray showing shotgun pellets and an "old" bullet.

findings "were considered consistent with the residuals of esophageal perforation by a bullet." The movement of the metallic foreign body through the gastrointestinal tract was followed with x-rays and the "missile" was passed per rectum. Spectrograph examination of the metallic piece revealed a composition of mercury, silver and copper. These elements suggested a similarity to metal used for dental fillings. In fact, a dental examination of the patient revealed bilateral molar restorations with a section of a restoration approximating the size of the "missile" missing.

Autopsy Artefacts

Artefacts may be introduced during the performance of an autopsy. Careless cutting of the tissues may obliterate the bullet tracks and the evaluation of the angle of fire may be rendered difficult. Similarly, the displacement of the bullet from one area to another in the body during an autopsy may affect conclusions about the direction of fire.

While sawing off the vault of the skull during autopsy, partial sawing and forceful pull of the cap sometimes lead to fractures of the skull. In an already fractured skull, the antemortem fracture caused by gunshot may be extended or additional fractures may be created. At times it may be impossible to differentiate a postmortem fracture from an antemortem one. Therefore, due care should be exercised if accurate documentation of a gunshot head injury is to be made.

Miscellaneous Artefacts

In the investigation of cases of gunshot wounds, the findings of unexpected bullets in the body is always a puzzle and may lead to false conclusions (Fig. 12-4). Here is an example of an "old" bullet in the body:

In a case of a severely burned body, x-rays showed a bullet in the posterior wall of the chest. This x-ray finding immediately raised suspicions of murder. However, when the bullet was localized and removed, it was found to be well wrapped with dense fibrous tissue.

In another case a "new" bullet formed an artefact:

A man shot himself in the right temple and the bullet was recovered from the brain. There was, however, another bullet in the stomach. The scene investigation showed a row of beer cans in the man's backyard, used as targets. Part of the beer in the cans that had bullet holes had been consumed. It is surmised that the man drank beer from each can he shot successfully and "drank" a bullet with the beer.

Injuries such as puncture wounds and lacerations may resemble exit and entrance wounds. Therefore, every care should be taken to identify such injuries correctly.

Importance of Identifying the Artefacts

In medicolegal cases misinterpretations may turn out to have disastrous effects. If the pathologist is to avoid mistakes in the performance of a medicolegal necropsy, particularly in an instance in which homicide is a possibility, he should be aware of artefacts. If an autopsy finding is so important that it may make the difference between the freedom or imprisonment, or the life and death of someone, it is the duty of the pathologist to interpret that finding correctly. He must realize that misinterpretations may lead to:

1. A wrong cause of death
2. A wrong manner of death
3. Undue suspicions of criminal offense
4. A halt in the investigation of a homicide or non-detection of a murder

5. Unnecessary spending of time and effort as a result of misleading findings
6. Miscarriage of justice in civil suits

It must also be stressed that a mistake made by a pathologist in the interpretation of an artefact may haunt him later in the court as counsel attempts to shake his testimony as a pathologist because of the error.

REFERENCES

1. Burton, C.: The case of the mysterious missile. Journal of Trauma, 9:257, 1969.
2. Dorland's Illustrated Medical Dictionary. ed. 24. Philadelphia, W. B. Saunders, 1965.
3. Fatteh, A.: Artefacts in forensic pathology. *In* Wecht, C. (ed.): Legal Medicine Annual, 1972. New York, Appleton-Century-Crofts, 1972.

13

Unusual Weapons, Ammunitions
and Wounds

Unusual gunshot wounds may result from weapons not conventionally sold as firearms. For instance, tear gas pen guns, zip guns, tear gas shells and toy guns may cause unusual injuries. Puzzling situations may arise when unusual ammunition is used or a particular type of ammunition is not used in a traditional way. On rare occasions, one may see unusual patterns of injury because of a defective weapon, faulty ammunition or improper use of these. Also, unusual human behavior may account for situations that are out of the ordinary. Recognition and proper interpretation of unusual wounds is important. A variety of unusual firearms and ammunitions will be discussed and some cases of unusual wounds presented in this chapter.

UNUSUAL WEAPONS

Tear Gas Pen Guns

Tear gas pen guns, now classified as firearms in the U.S., are commonly used for personal defense. Tear gas, Chloro-acetophenone, is an irritant and produces lacrimation and irritation of skin and respiratory tract. Many instances of injury to the eyes have been reported.[16,19] Hand injuries may also be caused by these guns.[1] If the shot is fired at contact range, the wad entering the body may cause inflammatory foreign body reaction or fatal injury.[28]

In an excellent article, Stahl and Davis have given details of two deaths caused by tear gas pen guns.[27] In one of their cases, a man who was threatened by his acquaintance shot the assailant in the eye with a 0.38 caliber tear gas fountain pen gun loaded with a conventional pistol cartridge. The copper-jacketed bullet penetrated the skull and perforated the right temporal and occipital lobes of the brain. Death occurred 3½ hours after the shooting. The pen gun was such that it could fire either 0.38 caliber tear gas ammunition or 0.38 caliber metallic cartridges.

In another instance, a 42-year-old man shot himself in the neck under the chin with a 0.38 caliber tear gas pen gun. The bullet travelled up into the cranium and was found lodged in the right frontal lobe of the brain. The man had left a suicide note. Powder residue was observed on his left second finger.

These authors have also described a case in which a serviceman sustained a gunshot wound of the abdomen as a result of accidental firing of a 0.22 caliber tear gas pen gun loaded with 0.22 caliber long-rifle hollow point ammunition. The bullet entered the abdominal cavity, perforated the stomach and penetrated the liver. The serviceman recovered from the effects of the injuries.

A study describing injury potential of tear gas pen guns reloaded with primer, powder, BB shot pellets and wads to simulate shotgun shells has been published.[11] The results indicate that the average velocity of pellets discharged is about 584 feet per second and that the shot is capable of causing sublethal and lethal injuries in experimental animals at distances from contact to 18 inches.

Another recent report contains ballistic studies and lethal potential of tear gas pen guns.[12] A set of ten illegal pen guns capable of firing 0.22 through 0.44 caliber magnum pistol or revolver cartridges and 0.270 caliber rifle cartridges was obtained by the authors from the Bureau of Alcohol, Tobacco, and Firearms of the U.S. Department of Treasury for test fires and other studies. The results of their investigations include observations about the velocity, range of accuracy, impact kinetic energy, and gelatin block penetrability of bullets fired by these pen guns.

Zip Guns

A zip gun is a crude homemade single-shot firearm. Any objects that come handy to the maker are used in constructing a zip gun. Car radio telescoping antenna is commonly used to make a 0.22 caliber barrel. Zip gun barrels do not have rifling striae. The gun bore is usually larger than the cartridge. Consequently, the cartridge rests loosely in the bore. The markings on fired bullets and cartridges are unusual. They may result from projections at the muzzle and within the barrel, but no rifling marks are seen. Whenever unusual markings are observed on a fired bullet or cartridge case the use of a zip gun should be suspected. Various problems encountered in the investigation of a shooting with a zip gun and identifying characteristics of zip guns and ammunition fired with zip guns have been discussed at length by Koffler.[14]

Cap-Firing Pistols

These too are crude creations made to fire live ammunition. A toy cap pistol is modified to make it fire a 0.22 caliber rimfire cartridge. A cap-firing pistol is usually a light metal casting held together by rivets. This is converted to a weapon capable of firing live ammunition by removing the barrel rivet and inserting a piece of car radio antenna or some other metal tubing and providing a firing pin. The firing pin is made by drilling a hole in the hammer and screwing in a self-tapping screw. The hammer may be strengthened by wrapping rubber bands around the frame and the back of the hammer.

The Mattel "Shootin' Shell" guns and replica toy derringer pistols are variations of the cap pistol.[15]

The cap-firing conversions are capable of causing fatal injuries. Di Maio and Spitz have reported a case in which a 15-year-old white male committed suicide by shooting himself in the temple with a toy derringer.[6] A portion of radio antenna had been inserted in the upper barrel of the pistol.

The injuries caused by cap-firing pistols have no characteristic features. The fired bullets lack rifling marks.

Stud Guns

Stud guns are tools used to fire metal studs into wood, concrete and steel. They utilize special cartridges ranging from 0.22 to 0.38 caliber. Stud guns are capable of causing severe injuries because of their high penetration power.[26]

Injuries from stud guns are rare. Only one report of death from a stud gun injury could be found in the literature.[6] In this case, a 50-year-old man was found dead in bed with a wound of the forehead. A stud gun containing a fired 0.22 caliber cartridge was found near the body. At autopsy, a perforating wound of the skull and brain was seen. The stud fired from the gun was embedded in the wall behind the man's head.

Weapons with Microgrooves

In most of the rifled weapons there are four to eight lands and grooves. In recent years a new system of rifling has been developed for 0.22 caliber rifles. It consists of microgrooves, numbering 15 to 20, in the barrel. The grooves have rounded edges instead of traditional square edges. These round edges make the matching of the bullets difficult. However, from the examination of the bullet it is not difficult to say that it was fired from a rifle with microgroove rifling.[20]

Toy Guns

Accidental discharge of firearms is not uncommon. In most instances the bullet fired is intended to be shot from the gun that fires it. This is not always so, however, as illustrated above by the misuse of tear gas pen guns. Haddad and his colleagues reported an unusual instance of accidental discharge of live ammunition by a toy "cork" gun.[9] The gun was loaded by the friend of the victim with a 0.38 caliber revolver bullet. When the gun was fired, the bullet exploded and caused a gunshot wound of the abdomen.

Air Rifles

Air rifles have low velocity and are said to be safe weapons. They have, nevertheless, the potential to cause serious injury and even death. Death may result if the shot enters the brain through the eye or if such an injury is associated with serious complications. Polson has reported a case in which a boy was shot in the eye with an air rifle and died from brain injuries.[21]

Recent literature records a case of an accidental death by an air rifle reported by Chandu Lal and Subrahmanyam.[4] In this case, accidental firing of an air rifle resulted in the victim's being hit by a pellet under the eye. Although the pellet, measuring 0.7 cm in length and 0.5 cm in diameter, did not perforate the eyeball it travelled through the floor of the orbit to the cavernous sinus of the opposite side. Death was from hemorrhage and aspiration of blood.

UNUSUAL AMMUNITIONS

Frangible Bullet

Frangible bullets were developed for use in shooting galleries and to kill cattle. In the ammunition used for the gallery, the cartridges are composed of 15 grains of powdered iron and 29 grains of powdered lead with an organic binder. The ones used for stunning and killing cattle are composed of powdered iron with an organic binder. The bullets are available in 0.22 caliber size. The brand names, weights and velocities of various commercially available frangible bullets are presented in Table 13-1.

Fatalities from frangible bullet wounds are extremely rare. Graham et al. have reported a death from a 0.22 caliber frangible bullet.[8] In that case an 18-year-old Negro youth was spinning the cylinder and pulling the trigger of a revolver pointing at his right temple when the gun fired. He died four hours later. At autopsy a contact gunshot wound was seen

Table 13-1.   Commercially Available Frangible Bullets

Brand Name	Weight (in grains)	Velocity (feet per second)
Winchester Short Spatterpruf	29	1045
Western Short Kant-Splash	29	1045
Remington Short Spatter-Less	29	1045
Peters Short Krumble Ball	29	1045
Winchester Num-Rite Super	15	1625
Winchester Short Spatterpruf	15	1710
Western Short Kant-Splash	15	1710
Remington Short Spatter-Less	15	1710
Winchester Num-Rite Short	15	1710
Winchester Num-Rite Regular	15	2200
Winchester Num-Rite Magnum	20	2650

in the right temple region. The bullet perforated the brain, and one of its fragments weighing 26 grains was retrieved. This was brittle and hard and was readily attracted by a magnet. The irregularity of the fragment made it impossible to make comparison tests.

Frangible bullets deform and fragment easily after impact and hence they are usually unsuitable for identification by comparison microscopy. The authors who reported the above fatality conducted experiments to determine the degree of penetration, fragmentation and suitability of fired bullets for comparison microscope identification. They fired shots in calf heads for this study. They noted wide variation in the degree of penetration and fragmentation of these bullets and all test bullets were such that comparison tests were not possible.

Bird Shot

Cartridges loaded with No. 12 shot are available in 0.22 caliber size. These are meant to be used for pest control. They are loaded with wadding and about 150 pellets, each 0.05 inch in diameter. They could be loaded in 0.22 caliber pistols and revolvers. They are low velocity cartridges and do not cause significant injuries unless they are fired from close range.

Fatalities from bird shot wounds are extremely rare. Di Maio and Spitz have reported a homicide involving a bird shot cartridge.[5] The victim was shot in the temple region from a distance of less than 6 inches but not at contact range.

In the following case investigated by this author the victim sustained wounds in the head with an unusual combination of 0.22 caliber shot cartridge with No. 12 shot and a 0.22 caliber cartridge containing a bullet. The man was shot either with two different guns or with one

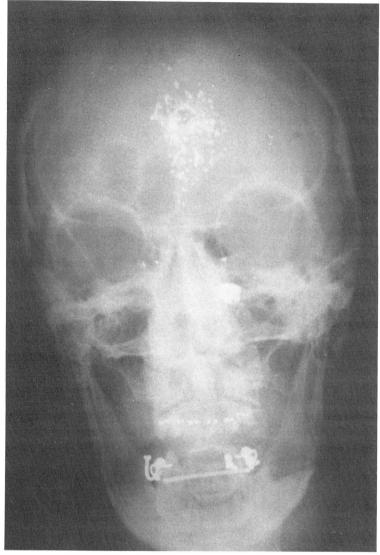

Fig. 13-1. X-ray showing bird shot pellets and a 0.22 caliber missile.

weapon loaded with bird shot cartridges and regular 0.22 caliber cartridges containing bullets.

A 50-year-old man was found dead lying face up on the living room floor by his wife when she came home. The house had been ransacked. The weapon was not found.

External examination of the body revealed a contact gunshot wound, ¼ inch

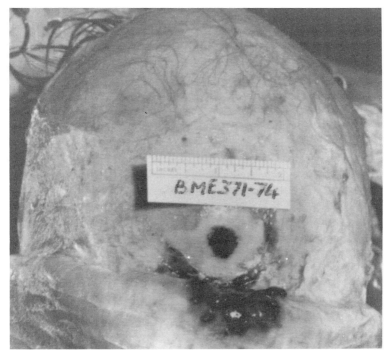

Fig. 13-2.   Hole in the skull caused by No. 12 bird shot.

in diameter, in the center of the forehead. There was smoke, flame and gunpowder effect around the wound in an area ¾ inch in diameter (see Fig. 11–5). Another contact gunshot wound, ¹/₆ in diameter with shot soiling in an area ⁵/₁₆ inch in diameter was present in the center of the back of the neck. There was an abrasion, ⁵/₁₆ × ³/₁₆ inch, in the lower margin of this wound. X-rays of the head showed numerous shot pellets in the frontal lobes and a bullet lodged in the bone in the left middle fossa (Fig. 13-1). Internal examination showed a round hole ⁷/₁₆ inch in diameter in the frontal bone at the point of entry of bird shot (Fig. 13-2). Many pellets and a miniature wad were retrieved from the medial aspects of the frontal lobes together with a deformed 0.22 caliber bullet which was lodged in the middle fossa. The bird shot had travelled directly backwards and the bullet, which had entered the back of the neck, had travelled forwards, upwards and slightly to the left.

Blank Cartridges

A blank cartridge is a cartridge case with primer, gunpowder and wadding but no bullet. Such cartridges are used in army rifles for practice maneuvers, in starter pistols for sporting events and in pistols fired on stage. The propellant in these cartridges is fast burning and can produce considerable noise.

When blank cartridge shots are fired from a long distance they are harmless. They can, however, cause serious injuries from close ranges. Experimental work indicates that shots fired from a distance of one inch can cause tears in the skin and subcutaneous tissues and at contact range they could cause wounds up to 2½ inches deep.[25]

Blank cartridges are capable of causing fatal injuries. Wounds resulting from discharge of a blank cartridge from a weapon held in contact against the palm of the hand have proved fatal.[7] A fatality of a 14-year-old boy by blank cartridge shot is reported. In this case a shot fired from a pistol containing a 0.32 caliber blank cartridge at contact range in the precordial region resulted in a hole through the skin, intercostal muscles, pericardium and right ventricle, and the boy died of hemopericardium.[7]

Tear Gas Shells

In 1967, Ramu reported from India a death from tear gas shell.[22] A 10-year-old boy was killed when police tried to disperse a crowd with special artillery shells containing chloro-acetophenone fired in a barrage. At autopsy, an exploded tear gas shell, 7½ inches long and ¾ inch in diameter, was found lodged in the neck. The wound of entry was behind and below the right ear and the wound of exit on the right side of the front of the neck. The shell was in the track of the wound with its base in the entrance wound and its nose end protruding from the exit wound.

Tandem Bullets

A bullet propelled out of the chamber of a gun may remain stuck in the barrel either due to a defect in the weapon or due to faulty ammunition. If the trigger is pulled again the second bullet may propel the bullet stuck in the barrel and both bullets may travel together. Such bullets are called tandem bullets. Usually the two bullets are stuck together when they leave the muzzle and cause one entrance wound. They may, however, separate within the body or before they hit the target.

In a case described by one team of investigators, two bullets entered the temple area in tandem causing one entrance wound but causing two perforations, one inch apart, in the cranium on the opposite side.[7]

In another case the bullets apparently separated before they hit the victim.[25] One bullet hit the victim in the chest and the other entered the body at the inner angle of the right eye. The bullets were fired from a defective 0.38 caliber revolver.

Even if the tandem bullets are fired at contact range, the usual features caused by flame, smoke and gunpowder may be diminished or absent and the wound may appear as if caused by long-range fire. This is because the propelling force of the second bullet is directed backwards due to obstruction caused by the first bullet impacted in the barrel.

Lowbeer described a case of tandem bullets in which the contact wound caused by the bullets joined together showed only slight blackening of the subcutaneous tissues.[17] Muzzle imprint was, however, present around the bullet wound.

When the two fused bullets are separated, the nose end of the second bullet will show a fitting impression caused by the base of the first bullet. Another important feature that the tandem bullets show is that they have matching markings caused by the lands and grooves of the barrel.

KTW Ammunition

This new form of ammunition is designed for penetrating the body of an automobile or the engine block. It is available in several pistol calibers including 0.30 carbine. The cartridges are loaded with metal-piercing teflon-coated tungsten alloy bullets that have a half-jacket of gilding metal. The half-jacket serves as a rotating band and causes the bullet to spin. A commonly used KTW ammunition is the 0.38 Special, which has a muzzle velocity of 700 feet per second.

The injuries caused by KTW ammunition do not have special characteristics. It is important to remember, however, that the half-jacket may get separated from the bullet during its course through the body. The bullet may exit from the body but the half-jacket may not. In view of the presence of an exit wound, the jacket may not be searched for. Since only the jacket bears the barrel markings, identification of the gun will not be possible if the half-jacket is not recovered from the body. Therefore, if the use of KTW ammunition is suspected, x-rays of the body should be made, even if an exit wound is present, so that the half-jacket is not missed.

Super Vel Ammunition

The Super Vel Corporation has recently developed a new loading for the 0.38 Special. It consists of a light-weight, semi-jacketed bullet with a muzzle velocity of 1370 feet per second. This ammunition has replaced the 0.38 Special in many police departments because of its higher muzzle velocity and muzzle energy. Two types of Super Vel bullet are available: a hollow-point and a flat nose soft-point.

The Super Vel bullets cause skin wounds similar to those caused by the 0.38 Special. However, the bullet tracks within the body are larger and the tissue damage greater with the Super Vel bullets. The hollow-point Super Vel has greater destructive effect than the flat nose soft-point.

Ball Powder

Ball powder, a form of smokeless powder, was introduced by Winchester-Western just prior to World War II. The grains of ball powder are in the form of spheres and not cylinders or flakes as in other smokeless gunpowders. The use of ball powder has increased in recent years. Many of the pistol cartridges produced by Winchester-Western contain ball powder. By comparison with other smokeless powders, however, the use of ball powder is not common. For the purpose of exclusion this is important. For instance, if ammunition loaded with ball powder is used and the shot is fired from close or intermediate range, it may be possible to exclude the use of other powders from the examination of the wound. The skin surface and the subcutaneous tissues may reveal spheres of unburnt powder indicating the use of ball powder. Even if the shot is fired from long range, it may be possible to conclude from the examination of the bullet that ball powder was used. This is because ball powder frequently causes several small pockmarks on the base of the bullet.

A Marble as a Bullet

In a case cited in Taylor's Principles and Practice of Medical Jurisprudence (1965) a young man who wanted to shoot himself used the case of an Italian iron in which he made a touch-hole.[24] Using a marble for the bullet, he fired it into his mouth.

A Bolt as a Projectile

A case of a fatal gunshot wound of the chest has been described by Chandra Gowda in which a bolt was used instead of pellets in a muzzle-loading shotgun.[3]

UNUSUAL GUNSHOT WOUNDS

Multiple (More than Two) Suicidal Gunshot Wounds

Multiple gunshot wounds are usually but not necessarily homicidal. In the previous chapter, fourteen cases of suicidal gunshot wounds, each with two wounds, have been described. On rare occasions, cases with more than two suicidal gunshot wounds are encountered.

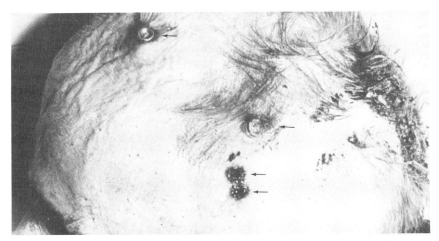

Fig. 13-3. Four suicidal gunshot wounds of the head (Courtesy of Hobart Wood, M.D.).

Wood investigated an unusual case with four suicidal gunshot wounds in the head:*

When an elderly recluse was not seen up and about in his apartment for a few days, his neighbors summoned police to investigate. On breaking open his apartment door, he was found lying on the bed. An old 0.32 caliber revolver was found on his body with very old ammunition. There were four gunshot wounds on the head (Fig. 13–3). Two penetrated the scalp, one penetrated the skull and one entered the cranium. He had suffered from severe arthritis and in a suicide note that he had left he cited poor health as the reason for taking his own life.

Mason and his associates have documented details of a case in which a 74-year-old man committed suicide by shooting himself four times in the head and once in the chest.[18] The man, who had become increasingly despondent, was found dead in the driver's seat of his station wagon. His pistol was found lying on the front passenger seat. There was a suicide note in his coat pocket. Examination of the body showed four contact gunshot wounds in the head—one in the right temple, two above the right ear and one above and posterior to the right ear. There was also a contact gunshot wound slightly to the left of the center of the chest. X-rays of the skull showed four flattened and deformed missiles at the points of entrance gunshot wounds in the head. None of the bullets had penetrated the skull. The bullet that entered the chest perforated the heart, diaphragm and the stomach, and death resulted from hemopericardium. The pistol found in the car was a 0.32 caliber Omega

---

*Wood, H.: Personal communication, 1972.

revolver containing six spent cartridges. All cartridges had ruptured. Examination of these cartridge cases revealed that they were 0.32 caliber Colt Short. They were not the proper ammunition for 0.32 caliber Omega revolver, which is chambered for 0.32 S & W Long cartridges. Thus, the improper ammunition resulted in lower muzzle velocity causing superficial head wounds.

Gonzales and his colleagues have reported two cases with multiple suicidal gunshot wounds.[7] In one, the victim inflicted three closely placed contact gunshot wounds in the region of the left upper quadrant of the abdomen and one contact wound in the right temple region. A 0.32 caliber revolver was used. Three bullets were recovered from the left posterior chest wall. The gunshot wound of the head was considered to be fatal. In another case, the victim shot himself five times in the right temple region. All bullets perforated the skull but none injured the brain; nevertheless, he died from sepsis several days after the shooting.

In a case reported in Glaister's Medical Jurisprudence and Toxicology (1973) the victim used a small caliber revolver to commit suicide.[23] He fired five shots at contact range in an area 3 inches in diameter over the third and fourth intercostal space 1½ inches from midline.

Fatal Gunshot Wound of Fetus

Gunshot wounds of the pregnant uterus are rare. The English literature included 39 cases up to 1960.[2] In the last decade, additional cases have been reported, and the total number in 1969 was fifty.[29]

In the case described by Beattie and Daly, a 20-year-old primigravida sustained a bullet wound to the abdomen when a 0.22 caliber pistol, accidentally dropped, fired. The bullet perforated the uterus, the entrance wound being 8 cm to the right of midline and the exit 6 cm to the left of midline. At the time of surgical exploration it appeared that the bullet had probably missed the uterine cavity. The surgeon, therefore, chose to allow the fetus to remain intact. After the operation, however, no fetal heart sounds were heard, and one week after the shooting incident the mother spontaneously delivered a macerated male infant weighing three pounds.

Apart from accidental shooting injury of the fetus, the unborn child may sustain a gunshot wound if the mother attempts to commit suicide or if she is a victim of a criminal shooting.

A case of a fatal gunshot wound of a fetus, inflicted by the mother, has been reported by Kloss.[13] In this case, a married woman with a year-old child was 17 weeks pregnant. When she learned about her pregnancy, she became agitated and appeared convinced that because of her economic problems and poor home conditions she could not afford another child. She considered several ways of procuring an abortion but did not try any. When she was 20 weeks pregnant she shot herself by placing a rifle against her abdomen, succeeding in shooting the fetus "only after the third attempt." Surgical intervention saved the mother's life, but the fetus was dead from a through-and-through gunshot wound of the head. A psychiatrist's evaluation indicated that the woman's "attempt at procuring the abortion was also an attempt to take her own life."

A medicolegally interesting case of criminal abortion by gunshot has been described.[29] In this case, a woman, 32 weeks pregnant, was shot by her friend with a 0.22 caliber revolver. The friend had fired several test shots into stacks of paper of different thicknesses using several types of ammunition, in preparation for inducing abortion by shooting the fetus in utero. The bullet entered in the midline 3 cm below the umbilicus ending up in the head of the fetus which was delivered dead by Caesarian section.

Recently this author investigated the following unusual case.

A young Negro woman about 25 weeks pregnant was among eight other women involved in an argument in front of a bar. She got shot by one of the women with a 0.22 caliber pistol and was rushed to a hospital. An exploratory laparotomy was done and the uterus, which showed a through-and-through bullet wound in the lower segment, was removed with the fetus and the adnexal tissues. During its course the bullet clipped the umbilical cord and caused a "slap" wound on the front of the left leg of the fetus. When delivered the newborn was gasping. The physicians put the newborn on a respirator within minutes of delivery. It died, however, after 23 hours. The mother recovered without complications.

On the basis of the autopsy findings the immediate cause of death was listed as "Gunshot wound of the umbilical cord and the left leg while in utero" with "prematurity" as unrelated contributory cause. A Florida statute provides that "The wilful killing of an unborn quick child, by any injury to the mother of such child which would be murder if it resulted in the death of such mother, shall be deemed manslaughter. . . . "

In view of this law the death of the newborn was classified as "'homicide.'"

Unusual War Wound

Hyde reported a case of an unusual wound sustained by a United States soldier in Vietnam.[10] The young man and his patrol were attacked by hostile small-arms fire when he was hit by enemy fire. He sustained a through-and-through bullet wound of the left elbow. In addition, the soldier had a superficial wound of the right thigh involving the skin and subcutaneous fat. This wound showed "powder burns on the edges of the wound and innumerable grains of unburned gunpowder in the wound." There was a ragged base of an M-16 cartridge with intact primer in the soldier's right trouser pocket. It was surmised that the superficial wound of the thigh was caused when an enemy bullet struck the ammunition in the soldier's pocket and detonated the cartridge.

REFERENCES

 1. Adams, J. P., Fee, N. and Kenmore, P. I.: Tear Gas Injuries. A Clinical Study of Hand Injuries and an Exprimental Study of Its Effects on Peripheral Nerves and Skeletal Remains in Rabbits. J. Bone Joint Surg., *48A*:436, 1966.
 2. Beattie, J. F. and Daly, R. F.: Gunshot Wound of the Pregnant Uterus. Amer. J. Obst. & Gynec., *80*:1, 1960.
 3. Chandra Gowda, B. C.: A bolt as a projectile—Report of a case: Forensic Science, *1*:107, 1972.
 4. Chandu Lal, R. and Subrahmanyam, B. V.: Accidental Death by Air Rifle. Forensic Sci., *1*:441, 1972.
 5. Di Maio, V. J. M. and Spitz, W. U.: Injury by Birdshot. J. For. Sci., *15*:396, 1970.
 6. ———: Variations in wounding due to unusual firearms and recently available ammunition. J. For. Sci., *17*:377, 1972.
 7. Gonzales, T. A., Vance, M., Helpern, M. and Umberger, C. J.: Legal Medicine, Pathology and Toxicology, ed. 2. New York, Appleton-Century-Crofts, 1954.
 8. Graham, J. W., Petty, C. S., Flohr, D. M. and Peterson, W. E.: Forensic Aspects of Frangible Bullets. J. For. Sci., *11*:507, 1966.
 9. Haddad, R., Zahr, L. A., Khuri, S. and Harrison, T. S.: Medical Intelligence: Accidental Discharge of Live Ammunition by a Toy "cork" Gun with Associated Gunshot Wound of the Abdomen. J. of Trauma, *11*:793, 1971.
10. Hyde, H.: An Unusual Wound in Vietnam. S. Dakota J. Med., *21*:47, 1968.
11. Jones, S. R., Besant-Matthews, P. E., Williams, F. J. and Stahl, C. J.: Injury potential of a reloaded tear gas pen gun. J. For. Sci., *19*:812, 1974.
12. Jones, S. R., Stahl, C. J. and Harriman, J. J.: Ballistic studies and lethal potential of tear gas pen guns firing fixed metallic ammunition. J. For. Sci., *20*:261, 1975.
13. Kloss, M.: Fatal Gunshot Wound of Fetus Inflicted by the Mother. Aust. N.Z. J. Obstet. Gynaec. *4*:125, 1964.
14. Koffler, B. B.: Zip guns and crude conversions—Identifying characteristics and problems. J. Crim. Law, Criminology and Police Sci., *60*:520, 1969.
15. ———: Zip guns and crude conversions—Identifying characteristics and problems. J. Crim. Law, Criminology and Police Sci., *61*:115, 1970.
16. Levine, R. A. and Stahl, C. J.: Eye Injury Caused by Tear-Gas Weapons. Amer. J. Ophthal., *65*:497, 1968.
17. Lowbeer, L.: An Unusual Gunshot Wound of the Head. J. For. Sci., *6*:88, 1961.
18. Mason, M. F., Rose, E. and Alexander, F.: Four Non-Lethal Head Wounds Resulting from Improper Revolver Ammunition: Report of a Case. J. For. Sci., *12*:205, 1967.
19. Midtbo, A.: Eye Injury from Tear Gas. Acta Ophthal. (Kobenhavn), *42*:672, 1964.
20. Petty, C. S.: Firearms injury research. The role of the practicing pathologist. Am. J. Clin. Path., *52*:277, 1969.

21. Polson, C. J.: The Essentials of Forensic Medicine, ed. 2. London, Pergamon, 1956.
22. Ramu, M.: Death Due to a Tear Gas Shell: Report of a Case. J. For. Sci., 12:383, 1967.
23. Rentoul, E. and Smith, H.: Glaister's Medical Jurisprudence and Toxicology. Edinburgh, Churchill Livingstone, 1973.
24. Simpson, C. K. (ed.): Taylor's Principles and Practice of Medical Jurisprudence. London, J & A. Churchill, 1965.
25. Spitz, W. and Fisher, R. S. (eds.): Medicolegal Investigation of Death. Springfield, Charles C Thomas, 1973.
26. Spitz, W. U. and Wilhelm, R. M.: Stud gun injuries. J. For. Med., 17:5, 1970.
27. Stahl, C. J. and Davis, J. H.: Missile Wounds Caused by Tear-Gas Pen Guns. Amer. J. Clin. Path., 52:270–276, 1969.
28. Stahl, C. J., Young, B. C., Brown, R. J. and Ainsworth, C. A.: Forensic Aspects of Tear-Gas Pen Guns. J. For. Sci., 13:442, 1968.
29. Takki, S., Pollanen, L., Ertama, P. and Lehtonen, T.: Criminal Abortion by Gunshot. Annales Chirurgiae et Gynaecologiae Fenniae., 58:122, 1969.

14

Mysterious Missiles: Bullet Emboli

Recovery of a bullet fired at or in the body of the victim of a shooting is important. At the scene of the crime every effort must be made to find the bullets that have not hit the victim or that have gone completely through the body. The bullets may be embedded in the walls, floors, articles of furniture or they may fly out of the windows if the shooting occurs indoors. In cases of a shooting outdoors, a search of large areas should be undertaken. When necessary, a metal detector and portable x-ray machine should be employed to localize a bullet concealed from view at the scene of the crime. In murder cases, the police investigator should leave no stone unturned in the effort to retrieve all bullets.

The bullet may be retained in the body of the victim. Whether a living victim of a gunshot wound is being evaluated for treatment or a fatality from firearm wounds is investigated for medicolegal reasons, retrieval of such a bullet in the body may be necessary to identify the firearm used in the crime. In most cases, the bullet in the body is in the general direction of fire. However, in some instances, the bullet that enters the body and does not exit is not found at the expected location. The bullet will be found in an unexpected or unusual location in the following circumstances:

1. When it is deflected after it strikes a bone
2. When it exits from body orifices
3. When it enters the neck and drops into the trachea or main bronchi
4. When it is swallowed or carried away from the point of entry in the gastrointestinal tract by peristalsis
5. When it enters the heart or a blood vessel and gets carried with the blood stream to a distant location

DEFLECTED BULLETS

Deflection of the bullet after it strikes a bone in the body is not uncommon. Such a deflection can make recovery of the bullet difficult if

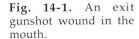

Fig. 14-1. An exit gunshot wound in the mouth.

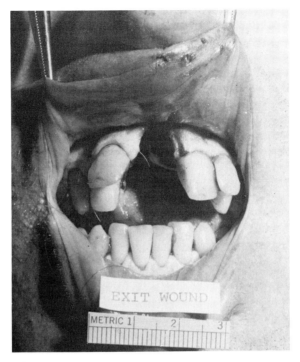

x-rays are not made. Occasionally, a bullet that hits a bone may travel around it. For instance, a bullet striking the skull may travel around the curvature of the skull under the scalp and may be found at an unexpected site. Similarly, a bullet striking a rib may travel under the skin along the outer aspect of the rib without entering the chest.

BULLETS EXITING FROM BODY ORIFICES

On rare occasions, bullets exit from body orifices. If the circumstances of death and the autopsy findings are not evaluated carefully, the whereabouts of the bullets exiting from body orifices may not be clear. The bullet that enters the head or neck may exit from the mouth or the bullet that penetrates the gastrointestinal tract may be passed per rectum if the victim of the shooting survives for a time. In such instances, a considerable amount of time may be expended in the search for a bullet if the possibility of its exit from one of the body orifices is not considered. The following case history illustrates this.

A 42-year-old man was shot by his wife with a 0.38 caliber handgun during an argument. The body showed an entrance wound in the neck, two in the front of the chest and one in the back. Only three exit wounds were seen initially, and multiple x-rays revealed no bullets in the body. After the possibility of bullet embolism was excluded, the body orifices were carefully examined. This revealed the exit of one of the bullets from the mouth. The bullet that had entered the right side of the neck had passed upwards and medially. It had perforated the tongue and exited from the mouth (Fig. 14-1).

Bullets in Air Passages

The bullet that enters the air passages may be coughed out or one that enters the mouth may be spat out. If such a bullet is not found at the scene of the shooting or in the vicinity of the victim, considerable confusion about its existence may be created. Peterson and Ruiz have reported a case in which a 0.38 caliber bullet was expectorated by a patient.[16] In that case, the victim, who was involved in a gun battle with police, sustained a gunshot wound of the chest. He complained of pain in the chest and shortness of breath. Chest x-rays revealed the bullet in the right hilar region. A bout of coughing caused expectoration of the bullet before planned surgery for its removal. The patient recovered from the effects of the gunshot wound.

Swallowed Bullets

The bullet that is swallowed or the one that enters the gastrointestinal tract at some point may be carried away by peristalsis. Such a bullet, if not already passed per rectum, may be found away from the point of entry.

EMBOLIZED BULLETS

Occasionally, a bullet gains access to the blood circulation and gets carried to a distant location in the body. This is called bullet embolization. If the bullet is not in the body in the general direction of fire and if there is no exit wound, a search of the arterial and venous systems, including the heart and lungs, should be made. Bullet embolization can cause difficulty in the search of the missile during an autopsy unless it is properly localized with the help of x-rays.

Bullet embolism is not common. A search of the literature by Keeley revealed 22 cases recorded during the period 1885 to 1951.[10] Since Keeley's review 22 additional cases have been recorded in the English literature.[4] Several more cases have remained unpublished.

In most cases of bullet embolization, the point of entry of the bullet is the aorta. Sometimes the site of entry is the heart or a vein. The site of lodgement of an embolized bullet or pellet may be in any part of the vascular system.

Emboli to Brain

No reports of bullet emboli in the brain could be found in the litera-ture. Shotgun pellets that enter the vascular system may be carried to the cerebral vessels because they are light in weight. Two cases of pellet embolism have been reported.

In one case, described by Piazza and Giast,[17] a 22-year-old man was accidentally shot by a friend while hunting. He was treated in the hospital for multiple buckshot wounds of the chest, face and arms. While he was in the hospital, he developed left hemiplegia. A plain x-ray of the skull revealed a buckshot pellet about 3 cm to the right and 1 cm above sella turcia. Right frontotemporal craniotomy and splitting of the Sylvian fissure revealed the presence of the pellet within the lumen of the right middle cerebral artery a few millimeters from its origin. The buckshot pellet was milked away and trapped below the level of the circle of Willis, to allow the blood to flow from the contralateral side.

In another case, reported by Gilder and Coxe,[8] a young man was shot at close range in the left side of the head and neck with a shotgun. One of the pellets embolized to the middle cerebral artery and the patient developed severe right hemiplegia and aphasia. Removal of the pellet resulted in clinical improvement of the patient.

Emboli to Neck and Upper Extremity

In 1951, Keeley reviewed the world literature on peripheral arterial bullet embolism.[10] Up to that time, no instances of bullet emboli in the upper extremities or in the neck were recorded but three cases have been published in recent years.

A report by Trimble describes a case of bullet embolus in the carotid artery.[20] In this case, a man had a gunshot wound in the right midclavicular line, just below the eighth rib, with no exit wound. There were no gunshot wounds in the neck. The bullet appeared to have entered the heart. It embolized and was palpable in the right side of the neck, over the carotid artery, which showed diminished pulsations. Nine days after the shooting, a 0.32 caliber bullet was removed from the common carotid artery. The lumen of the artery was occluded by the bullet with short segments of thrombosis, both proximal and distal to the embolized bullet.

An interesting case of 0.45 caliber bullet embolus, in the right axillary artery, has been reported.[18] In this case, a missile that entered the chest first passed through the right ventricular wall and then perforated the interventricular septum. From the left ventricle the slug embolized to the right axillary artery. The right wrist pulse was absent but im-mediately after arteriotomy and removal of the embolized bullet the pulse returned.

An occurrence of a pellet embolus in the brachial artery has been reported.[13] In this case, a 10-year-old boy was shot with an air rifle from a distance of 10 feet. The entrance wound was in the left fourth intercostal space just lateral to the sternal border. No exit wound was found. Fluoroscopic examination of the chest failed to show a metallic foreign body. The boy developed shortness of breath and pain in the right hand. No pulse could be felt at the right wrist. Examination of the right upper extremity led to the discovery of a palpable pellet in the brachial artery 5 cm from the apex of the axilla. Complete recovery followed surgical removal of the embolized pellet and closure of the entrance wound in the heart.

Emboli to Lungs

In 1948, Collins reported a case of self-inflicted gunshot wound of the chest in which the bullet first lodged in the interventricular septum of the heart.[3] When it became dislodged from there, it was carried into the right pulmonary artery. This embolization caused massive pulmonary infarction in the right lung.

In a case reported by Fatteh and Pate,[5] a man was found dead with a gunshot wound in the upper lateral aspect of the right shoulder. At autopsy the bullet was found to have travelled slightly to the left, downwards and backwards. It had perforated the upper lobe of the right lung and entered the heart through the anterolateral wall of the right ventricle. The bullet had been propelled from the ventricular cavity into the pulmonary trunk and carried as an embolus into the pulmonary artery to the lower lobe of the left lung from where it was retrieved.

Symbas and his colleagues reviewed the literature on projectile embolus of the lung in 1968.[19] They were able to find six reported cases of projectile embolus. In one case, the pulmonary embolus was a piece of shrapnel and in the other five cases it was a bullet. In each of these cases the projectile had entered the venous system distal to the right atrium. These authors gave details of three of their own cases. In one case, the bullet entered the venous system through the right atrium and embolized in the right posterior segmental artery; in another case, the missile entered the right thigh posteriorly and embolized in the first segment of the lingular artery; in the third case, the bullet injury was in the left flank with the embolized bullet impacted in the origin of the right anterior basilar segmental artery.

Emboli to Heart

Peripheral embolism of a bullet usually follows a gunshot wound of the heart or a major vessel. Embolization of a bullet following its entry into the venous system leads to its lodgement in the heart.

Padula and his colleagues indicate, "approximately twenty-six cases of embolization of bullets to the heart have been reported."[14] In eight of the cases, embolization of the bullet to the heart occurred immediately after the bullet entered the venous system. In ten cases, there was a delay, ranging from 2 days to 13 months, before embolization occurred. These authors have described an unusual case of delayed bullet embolism. A woman was admitted to the hospital after being shot in the abdomen. X-rays at that time showed the bullet in the pelvis. Laparotomy was performed, but the surgeon was unable to find the bullet in the pelvis. Nine days after admission, x-rays of the abdomen were repeated and they were interpreted as follows: "An absence of the bullet previously located anterior to the right lateral process of the first sacral segment. The bullet was, therefore, probably located in the pelvic colon and has since been passed." Six months after the shooting incident, the patient developed cough and fever. A chest x-ray was made and this revealed the presence of a bullet within the cardiac shadow. After a complete work-up, cardiotomy using cardiopulmonary by-pass was performed. The bullet was palpated within the myocardium adjacent to the annulus of the tricuspid valve near the orifice of the inferior vena cava. It was successfully removed and the patient made a complete recovery.

Morton and his associates encountered three cases in a period of four years in which bullets entered the venous system in the lower part of the abdomen and embolized to the right ventricle.[11] In each case, the bullet was removed utilizing cardiopulmonary by-pass and complete recovery followed.

Emboli to Iliac Artery

Bullets that enter the heart or the aorta most often tend to take a downward course towards the lower extremities. They may be found at the bifurcation of the abdominal aorta or be lodged in one of the iliac arteries.

This author has seen two cases in which the bullet was found at the bifurcation of the abdominal aorta. In one of these cases, a 0.32 caliber bullet entered the left ventricle of the heart and was found blocking the origin of the right common iliac artery. In another, a 0.38 caliber missile that had entered the thoracic aorta was found embolized in the lumen of the left common iliac artery at its origin. The review of 22 cases of bullet embolus by Di Maio and Di Maio includes three cases of bullet embolus in the iliac artery.[4] In two cases the bullet entered the heart and in the third the thoracic aorta. Blackford and his associates have recorded a case of low velocity pellet embolism to the internal iliac artery with the point of entry in the circulation clinically thought to be in the right pulmonary vein.[1]

Emboli to Femoral Artery

The reviews of the subject of bullet embolism by Keeley (1951) and by Di Maio and Di Maio (1972) indicate that the site of lodgement of a bullet embolus is predominantly a lower extremity. In the review of 22 cases by Keeley, there were 14 cases with bullet emboli in the left femoral and iliac arteries and two cases with emboli in the right femoral and iliac arteries. Of the 22 cases of lower extremity embolus reviewed by Di Maio and Di Maio, 14 involved emboli to the right side and eight to the left. These authors have described six cases of bullet embolism; in all six of them, the site of embolus was the femoral artery.

In some of the reported cases, obstruction of the vessels had caused ischemic changes leading to gangrene of the limb. Often there are signs and symptoms of vascular insufficiency without gangrene. Sufficient blood may flow around a small bullet or there might be adequate collateral circulation to prevent ischemic changes. Occasionally, a branch of the femoral artery may be blocked resulting in no serious consequences. In the case described by Fatteh and his colleagues,[6] for instance, the embolized bullet blocked only the profunda femoris artery, a branch of the femoral artery (Fig. 14-2). No signs of ischemia were present in the extremity. In a living patient it is advisable to remove the arterial embolus as soon as possible. Severe ischemic changes may necessitate amputation of the extremity.[12]

Emboli to Popliteal and Tibial Arteries

A small-caliber bullet will travel as distally in the artery as the lumen of the vessel will permit. Cases are on record in which bullets have embolized to popliteal and tibial arteries.

Garzon and Gliedman described in 1964 a case in which a 16-year-old boy, with an entrance gunshot wound in the chest and no exit wound, was diagnosed by arteriogram to have an embolized bullet, 0.22 caliber, in the right popliteal artery.[7] He had mild weakness in the leg and absent pulsations below the site of lodgement of the bullet. The bullet had entered the circulation through the thoracic aorta.

In another instance of popliteal artery embolus, described by Dillard and Staple, the missile, 0.22 caliber, entered the aortic arch and became lodged at the point of branching of the left popliteal artery.[3] In this case too, the victim had tenderness of the calf muscles and absence of pulses in the branches of the popliteal artery.

Painter and Britt have described an additional case of popliteal artery embolism in which a 0.22 caliber missile fired from a pistol from close range entered the thoraco-abdominal aorta.[15] In this case normal chest x-rays, absence of exit wound and weakness of right popliteal pulse and

Fig. 14-2. An embolized bullet in the profunda femoris artery (Fatteh, A., et al.: Bullet embolus of right profunda femoris artery. J. For. Med., 4:139, 1968).

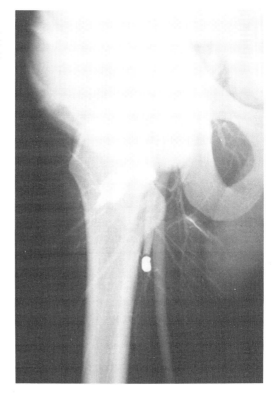

absence of right foot pulses led to the clinical diagnosis of bullet embolism.

Three cases of bullet embolism in the tibial artery have been reported. In the case described by Williams, a 0.22 caliber pistol fired at close range caused a gunshot wound just above the tip of the xiphoid.[21] The bullet was removed by arteriotomy from the posterior tibial artery. A 0.22 caliber bullet wedged tightly in the posterior tibial branch of the popliteal artery was similarly retrieved in the case described by Habein and Christensen.[9] In the case described by Trimble, a 0.22 caliber missile, which perforated the thoracic aorta, was localized radiographically and removed surgically from the left anterior tibial artery.[20]

CONCLUSION

Anytime one is confronted with a case of a mysterious missile, every effort should be made to solve the mystery. Careful search of the scene of the crime must be made; this may reveal the missing missile. The possibility of unusual pathways of the bullet within the body and of exit of the bullet from the body orifices must be kept in mind. If the bullet being searched for is suspected to be in the body of the victim, x-rays of the body, not excluding the extremities, should be taken.

REFERENCES

1. Blackford, J., Bowers, J. D., Taylor, P. M. and Heydinger, D. K.: Pellet embolism to the internal iliac artery. Am. J. Surgery, *118*:469, 1969.
2. Collins, D. H.: Bullet embolism: a case of pulmonary embolism following the entry of a bullet into the right ventricle of the heart. J. Path. & Bact., *60*:205, 1948.
3. Dillard, B. M. and Staple, T. W.: Bullet embolism from the aortic arch to the popliteal artery. Arch. Surg., *98*:326, 1969.
4. Di Maio, V. J. M. and Di Maio, D. J.: Bullet embolism: Six cases and a review of the literature. J. For. Sci., *17*:394, 1972.
5. Fatteh, A. and Pate, D. H.: Unusual bullet embolus. Brit. Med. J., *4*:609, 1972.
6. Fatteh, A., Shah, Z. A. and Mann, G. T.: Bullet embolus of the right profunda femoris artery. J. For. Med., *15*:139, 1968.
7. Garzon, A. and Gliedman, M. L.: Peripheral embolization of a bullet following perforation of the thoracic aorta. Ann. Surg., *160*:205, 1948.
8. Gilder, J. C. and Coxe, W. S.: Shotgun pellet embolus of the middle cerebral artery. J. Neurosurg., *32*:711, 1970.
9. Habein, H. C. and Christensen, R. K.: Bullet embolism from thorax to the popliteal artery. Rocky Mountain Med. J., *63*:35, 1966.
10. Keeley, J. L.: A bullet embolus to the left femoral artery following a thoracic gunshot wound. Case report and resume of peripheral arterial bullet embolism. J. Thoracic Surg., *21*:608, 1951.
11. Morton, J. R., Reul, G. J., Arbegast, N. R., Okies, J. E. and Beall, A. C.: Bullet embolus to the right ventricle—Report of three cases. Am. J. Surgery, *122*:584, 1971.
12. Movin, R., Russel, J. and Valle, A. R.: A migratory arterial foreign body. Am. J. Surgery, *91*:118, 1956.
13. Neerken, A. J. and Clement, F. L.: Air-rifle wound of the heart with embolization. JAMA, *189*:133, 1964.
14. Padula, R. T., Sandler, S. C. and Camishion, R. C.: Delayed bullet embolization to the heart following abdominal gunshot wound. Annals of Surgery, *169*:599, 1969.
15. Painter, M. W. and Britt, L. G.: Distal bullet embolism after gunshot wound of the chest: A case report. American Surgeon, *37*:106, 1971.
16. Peterson, T. A., and Ruiz, E.: The case of the tussive thief. JAMA, *204*:1974, 1968.
17. Piazza, G. and Gaist, G.: Occlusion of middle cerebral artery by foreign body embolus. Report of a case. J. Neurosurg., *17*:172, 1960.
18. Saltzstein, E. C. and Freearck, R. J.: Bullet embolism of the right axillary artery following gunshot wound of the heart. Annals of Surgery, *158*:65, 1963.

19. Symbas, P. N., Hatcher, C. R. and Mansour, K. A.: Projectile embolus of the lung. J. Thoracic & Cardiovascular Surgery, 5:97, 1968.
20. Trimble, C.: Arterial bullet embolism following thoracic gunshot wound. Annals of Surg., *168*:911, 1968.
21. Williams, D. J.: Embolization of a bullet to the posterior tibial artery following a gunshot wound of the thorax. J. Trauma, *4*:258, 1964.

15

Physical Activity Following Fatal Firearm Injury

In cases of gunshot wounds a question frequently asked is whether or not it is possible for a victim to perform purposeful activity after being shot. The extent of injury and the location of the wound are, of course, important factors. Notwithstanding the seriousness of the injuries, there is a great variation in the physical activity a victim of a gunshot wound can perform. Remarkable cases of volitional activity after serious head injury have occurred although the damage done might have been expected to have caused death almost instantly. It is possible for a victim of a gunshot wound of the heart to survive for a time and perform various activities, such as walking, running, climbing stairs and even driving a car, before collapsing. In this chapter several case histories are presented to illustrate the extent of physical activity that may be possible after sustaining gunshot wounds to different parts of the body.

WOUNDS OF THE BRAIN

The area of the brain injured by the gunshot blast has an important bearing on the degree of volitional activity. Bullet wounds of the brain usually involve the cerebrum. If a vital area such as the medulla, pons or the midbrain is shattered, death will be rapid. With damage to other areas of the brain, prolonged survival and variable degrees of activity are possible.

A case of suicide with a 0.45 caliber revolver illustrating unusual activity after extensive brain injury has been cited.[4] In this case a man shot himself under the chin. The bullet travelled upwards, passed through the left frontal and temporal lobes of the brain and exited through a hole 1¼ inches in diameter at the top of the head. The shot

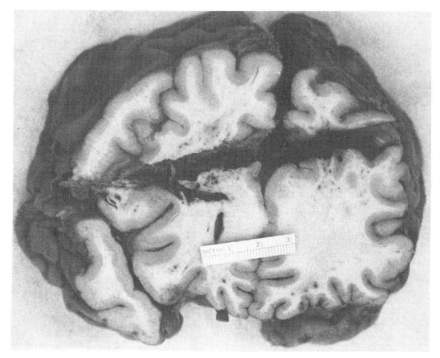

Fig. 15-1. A track within the brain substance caused by a 0.22 caliber missile.

blasted portions of bone and brain to the ceiling of the shelter in which the suicide took place. After shooting, the man walked around in snow, for at least 165 yards, and then walked across the road to his house. On arrival at home he spoke intelligibly to his maid, hung up his umbrella and overcoat, walked upstairs and collapsed. He lived for four hours after the estimated time of infliction of the gunshot injury.

A bullet wound of the brain is usually in the form of a cylindrical tunnel through the tissue. The diameter of the wound is invariably greater than the size of the bullet. The tissue in the margins of the track is ragged and hemorrhagic. Hemorrhage on the brain surface or within the brain matter is usually caused by laceration of arteries or venous sinuses. Shock from hemorrhagic and tissue damage curtails physical activity after shooting (Fig. 15-1).

A 31-year-old Negro male was shot in the left forehead region through a glass window as he was trying to break into a house. He ran a distance of about 50 feet and collapsed. He was dead when police arrived 15 minutes after the shooting. At autopsy a 0.32 caliber bullet lodged in the right occipital lobe was found

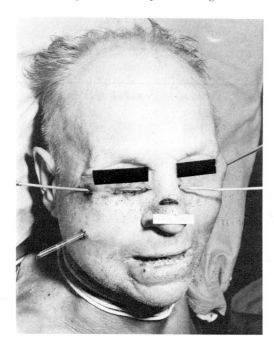

Fig. 15-2. Suicide by hanging. The victim shot himself three times before resorting to hanging.

to have caused a tunnel-like wound extending from the tip of the left frontal lobe to the tip of the right temporal lobe.

Occasionally a bullet fired in the head travels in such a direction that the brain is not injured. The victim in such an instance might suffer mild concussion and shock but may be able to perform various volitional acts.

A 75-year-old man was found hanging by a rope from a curtain rod in his living room. The doors of the apartment were locked on the inside. Gas had been turned on from the gas range in the adjoining kitchen. A typed will was tacked to the wall in the living room. A handgun was found approximately 12 feet away from the body on a night table in the bedroom. This was a suicide from hanging. However, the victim had attempted to take his life with a gun prior to hanging himself. A contact gunshot wound was found between the left eye and the left ear. The bullet had travelled slightly forward, downward and to the right. It had fractured the facial bones and exited from the center of the right cheek. Another entrance gunshot wound with associated powder stippling was present just below and to the right of the outer angle of the right eye. This bullet had travelled to the left and exited on the left side of the nose. A third bullet wound, a graze, with slight powder stippling was present on the front of the midportion of the nose. The bullet wounds had caused considerable bleeding and the scatter of the blood indicated that the man had walked around in the apartment after firing the shots (Fig. 15-2).

After injury the victim may perform voluntary or involuntary activity. While some activity may be a result of conscious effort, on the other hand, involuntary activity of which the victim is not aware may also be carried out after sustaining a gunshot wound of the head.

WOUNDS OF THE HEART

Penetrating and perforating wounds of the heart are serious injuries and the majority of them prove fatal in a short time. The survivability following a bullet injury of the heart and the extent of physical activity after the injury depend on the location of the bullet wound. Wounds of the auricles are the most rapidly fatal, wounds of the right ventricle come next and the wounds of the left ventricle are the least rapidly fatal. The thick muscle of the left ventricle, because of its power of contraction, may close the wound (and even lead to spontaneous healing) and produce hemostasis.

Vance has discussed three unusual bullet wounds of the heart showing attempts at healing.[5] In one instance, a 0.32 caliber bullet perforated the left lung and the pericardium and cut a tunnel in the surface of the heart without penetrating it. There was practically no hemorrhage in the pericardial cavity. Death resulted from a spinal cord injury seven days after the shooting. In another instance, a 0.25 caliber bullet perforated the pericardium, heart, and thoracic aorta, and penetrated the thoracic spine. The victim lived for eight days. At autopsy, a bullet wound was seen through the anterior surface of the right ventricle with perforations of the pulmonary artery, one of the pulmonary cusps, the left auricle and the thoracic aorta. The pericardial sac contained 250 cc of blood, the source of which was a recent separation of the edges of the right ventricular wound. In the third case described by this author, a bullet, causing injury of the heart through the right auricle was found lodged in the muscle of the right ventricle. The bullet track was scarred and the missile, a 0.28 caliber slug, was found enclosed in thick fibrous tissue. The gunshot wound had been sustained three years before death. The bullet injuries were incidental findings. Vance also mentions a case in which a 21-year-old man survived 24 hours despite being wounded in the left lung, the pericardium, the coronary venous sinus and both auricles by a 0.38 caliber bullet.

Winter has described a case of a through-and-through gunshot wound of the heart with recovery.[6] In this case, a 20-year-old man was shot by his wife with a 0.38 caliber pistol. After he was shot he was able to get up from bed, wrest the gun away from his wife, stagger outside and shout for help. He was taken to the hospital in a collapsed state, and

(Text continued on p. 209)

Table 15-1.   Physical Activity and Time of Survival
After Gunshot Injury

Case No.	Age, Sex and Race of Victim	Caliber of Bullet Causing Injury	Organs Injured and Type of Injury	Physical Activity After Injury	Time Between Injury and Death
1	25 NM	0.32	Through and through wound of aorta and left lung	Crawled 33 feet before collapse	Few minutes
2	8 NM	0.22	Through and through wound of heart	Staggered from second floor to the first	Twenty minutes
3	28 NF	0.32	Penetration of aorta, left lung and esophagus	Ran 45 feet	Thirty minutes
4	29 WM	0.22	Penetration of heart and right lung	Crawled 10 feet	One hour
5	33 NM	0.32	Penetration of heart, aorta, lung and liver	Crawled 7 feet	Short time
6	31 NM	0.22	Severance of right common cartoid artery and jugular vein	Crawled 12 feet	Six hours
7	36 NM	0.32	Penetration of heart, aorta and right lung	Ran out of apartment into street	Two hours

Table 15-1. Physical Activity and Time of Survival After Gunshot Injury (Continued)

Case No.	Age, Sex and Race of Victim	Caliber of Bullet Causing Injury	Organs Injured and Type of Injury	Physical Activity After Injury	Time Between Injury and Death
8	22 NM	0.32	Penetration of heart, lung and liver	Fell to ground, pulled his gun and fired at assailant	Twenty minutes
9	34 NM	0.32	Penetration of right lung; severance of intercostal artery and vein	Ran from second floor apartment to street and drove car five city blocks to hospital	More than one hour
10	31 NM	0.38	Perforation of heart and left lung	Crawled 55 feet	Several minutes
11	16 NM	0.32	Severance of superior mesenteric artery	Crawled about two city blocks	Fourteen hours
12	39 NM	0.32	Laceration of right lung; severance of intercostal vessels	Ran seven city blocks	Two hours

about 45 minutes after the shooting a thoracic surgeon commenced treatment. Thoracotomy revealed about 1000 cc of blood in the left chest cavity, an entrance gunshot wound in the right ventricle anterior to the descending branch of the left coronary artery and an exit wound in the posterolateral wall of the left ventricle. It appeared that the bullet had transversed the interventricular septum. The injuries in the heart were repaired. Postoperative recovery was uneventful.

Spitz and his colleagues have documented several cases with reference to physical activity after gunshot injury. These cases are summarized in Table 15-1.[2] Strassman has also reported five cases of gunshot injury to the heart.[3] In all his cases, the victims had engaged in various activities lasting up to 20 minutes after being wounded.

WOUNDS OF THE LUNGS AND OTHER ORGANS

Victims of gunshot wounds involving the lungs show variable volitional activity. The important factor in such cases is the extent and rapidity of hemorrhage. If a large artery or vein is perforated, profuse bleeding will occur rapidly, resulting in death in a few minutes. Even with rapid hemorrhage the victim may be able to walk or run several paces before shock from hemorrhage causes collapse. If a large vessel is not injured and bleeding is slow, the injured person may survive some hours or days. In the event of injury to a bronchus, death may occur from pneumothorax.

Injuries of the abdomen and the extremities are relatively simpler to interpret with reference to the victim's ability to perform physical acts after the shooting. Involvement of large vessels will cause rapid bleeding and shock. The amount and rapidity of blood loss will help the investigator formulate an opinion about the extent of physical activity that would be possible. Some instances of injury to lung, heart, aorta and other vessels are included in Table 15-1.

The effects of shotgun injuries are also variable. Contact and close-range shots will cause extensive tissue damage, hemorrhage and shock resulting in rapid death. With shots from greater ranges death may be delayed, and the victim may be able to perform various volitional acts. Fisher has described a case in which a 55-year-old man sustained a shotgun wound from a distance of 20 feet.[1] Two of the pellets perforated the abdominal aorta. With this injury he walked over a thousand yards and was able to get in a car by himself. He died on the way to a hospital within 20 minutes after the injury.

CONCLUSION

In a given case, an opinion about the extent of volitional activity after an injury must be guarded. It is unwise to assume that because the injury was grave, death must have been instantaneous. Involuntary and voluntary movements after extensive injuries to vital organs are possible. The victim may perform activities that appear incompatible with the injuries. This is particularly true for gunshot wounds of the brain and the heart. Every case must be judged individually after taking into consideration the autopsy findings and the circumstances surrounding the death.

REFERENCES

1. Fisher, R. S. *In* Spitz, W. U. and Fisher, R. S. (eds.): Medicolegal Investigation of Death Guidelines for the Application of Pathology to Crime Investigation. Chapter 10, Part 2, p. 245. Springfield, Charles C Thomas, 1973.
2. Spitz, W. U., Petty, C. S. and Fisher, R. S.,: Physical activity until collapse following fatal injury by firearms and sharp pointed objects. J. For. Sci., 6:290, 1961.
3. Strassman, G.: Uber Lebensdauer and Handlungsfahigkeit Schwerverletzter. Deut. Ztschr. f.d. Ges. Gerichtl. Med. 24:393, 1935.
4. Taylor, A. S. *In* Simpson, K. (ed.): Taylor's Principles and Practice of Medical Jurisprudence, ed. 11, vol. 1. Chapter 11. London, J. & A. Churchill, 1965.
5. Vance, B. M.: Three unusual cases of bullet wounds of the heart showing attempts at healing. Amer. J. Med. Sci., 169:872, 1925.
6. Winter, B.: Through and through gunshot wound of the heart with recovery. JAMA, 204:127, 1968.

16

Autopsy on the Body of a Prominent Public Figure

PREPARING FOR MEDICOLEGAL EMERGENCIES

The law enforcement agencies and the medical examiner's or coroner's office may be faced with the investigation of an emergency such as a mass disaster. In many places, plans are kept ready to deal with such a disaster. A medicolegal emergency of equally great national importance may be created by the assassination of a prominent public figure. One would hope that such a situation never occurs. However, in view of the series of assassinations of national figures in the past few years, a scheme of medicolegal investigation should be kept ready, just as is done for mass disasters, so that a complete and meticulous investigation can be accomplished.

In this chapter, an orderly consideration of various aspects of medicolegal investigation of the assassination of a prominent public figure is presented. Most assassinations of prominent persons have been committed with guns, thus the following discussion pertains to investigation of such a death caused by a firearm.

Since 1865, one out of every five U.S. Presidents has been assassinated and attempts have been made on the lives of three other Presidents—Theodore Roosevelt, Franklin D. Roosevelt and Harry S. Truman.[2] In addition, several other prominent persons have been the victims of gunfire. Factual accounts of the assassinations of Presidents Lincoln, Garfield, McKinley and Kennedy and of the assassinations of Robert F. Kennedy and Martin Luther King, Jr. have been published.[1,2] The autopsy on the body of President Abraham Lincoln was limited to the examination of the head. The report of that autopsy is reproduced in this chapter to provide a snapshot of medical science in transition. The autopsy investigations on the bodies of President John F. Kennedy and Senator Robert F. Kennedy, even though only five years apart in time, present a study in contrast. The autopsy on the body of President Kennedy was conducted in an environment of confusion and was incomplete. On the other hand, the postmortem examination of the body of Senator Kennedy was a beautifully organized effort ending with a widely acclaimed report. These reports are reproduced in this chapter with a few comments on each to bring out contrasting features. It is hoped that the general discussion that follows and these autopsy protocols will assist the reader in formulating plans for investigating a case of major importance.

PRE-TRAGEDY PREPARATIONS

Every medicolegal center should have plans to deal with a medicolegal situation caused by the assassination of a person of national or international prominence. The plans should include consideration of the place of autopsy, security of the location, availability of equipment, ease of communications with all the investigators, and dealings with the press.

Many investigators from various local and national organizations such as the Federal Bureau of Investigation, police departments and medical examiner's or coroner's office and several consulting investigators from throughout the country are likely to be involved in the investigation of the death of a national or international figure. The place selected for conducting the autopsy should be easily accessible so that there is no undue delay in securing the assistance of men from afar. The physical plant itself should be equipped with facilities for making x-rays.

The center should keep plans ready to install additional means of communications at short notice to deal with extra needs. The methods of handling inquiries from the news media should also be thought out in advance.

The person likely to be in charge of such a major investigation should make a list of investigators and consultants that he may want to invite for assistance and keep their addresses and telephone numbers ready.

If the place of tragedy is considered inadequate or unsuitable for conducting a proper investigation, arrangements should be made with the nearest facility that satisfies the criteria of being a satisfactory place for such an investigation. One must have a clear understanding of the legal questions concerning the authority to perform the autopsy and the removal of the body.

Personnel in the Autopsy Room

The medical examiner who is going to perform the autopsy should be in overall charge of the investigation in the autopsy room. He must determine, before commencing the autopsy, who should be present in the autopsy room. No unnecessary staff or unauthorized persons should be allowed to enter or pass through the autopsy room. In general, the staff in the autopsy room in a case of firearm death should include:

1. The forensic pathologist in charge of autopsy
2. Another forensic pathologist to assist the autopsy surgeon
3. A consulting pathologist experienced in the area of pathology of the organ injured
4. A representative from the Federal Bureau of Investigation
5. A representative from the local police department which has jurisdiction over the place of death.
6. A firearms examiner
7. A representative from the team of treating physicians (if the deceased was treated prior to death).
8. A mortuary assistant
9. A photographer
10. A medical secretary
11. A liaison officer

Forensic Pathologist in Charge of Autopsy.   He should be a competent pathologist with extensive experience in Forensic Pathology. If the tragedy occurs in an isolated community and the pathologist who has the legal jurisdiction over the case feels that he may not be able to handle the responsibility adequately, he should not hesitate to invite the assistance of a qualified pathologist and remain as an observer or assistant at the autopsy.

Assisting Pathologist.   He should also be a competent forensic pathologist with wide experience. He need not be from the office of the pathologist performing the autopsy. In fact, it is better to invite an experienced forensic pathologist from another place. He should preferably be one with special interest in medicolegal investigation of firearm deaths.

Consulting Pathologist.   A pathologist with special interest in pathology of the specific body area injured should also be available for consultation. For instance, in a case of gunshot wounds of the brain, a neuropathologist should be invited to render advice.

Representative from the FBI.   The Federal Bureau of Investigation will be involved in the investigation of a case of national importance. That Bureau has the responsibility of investigating various aspects of the case both nationally and internationally. Therefore, close cooperation with the Bureau is important. The presence of a representative from the FBI in the autopsy room will help in the exchange of information and could contribute to the interpretation of some of the findings.

Local Police Representative.   The local police department has an important task of coordinating various facets of the investigation. The findings of the autopsy will help them to evaluate the evidence and pursue certain lines of investigation. In addition, both the representative from the FBI and the one from the local police department can be of great assistance in collecting various articles of evidence. The police investigator from the local police department can also take charge of all the articles of evidence that the pathologist does not need to retain for his follow-up investigations, and turn them over to the proper authorities for further investigations.

Firearms Examiner. In every case of firearm fatality of national importance, the firearms examiner will be required to examine the firearm and any spent and unspent ammunition that may be found. Test firings will be necessary to determine the range of fire and to identify the weapon. The firearms examiner will be able to get a clear idea about the wounds on the body and the bullet holes in the clothes in their original state if he is present in the autopsy room. He may also be able to provide information about the gun and the ammunition and thus contribute to the interpretation of the injuries.

Representative from the Team of Physicians Rendering Treatment Before Death. If the victim survived for a time and was treated, it is important to have the details of treatment rendered. Information about the resuscitative efforts instituted before the victim was pronounced dead should be available before the autopsy is commenced. The best way to ensure the availability of the details of treatment is to ask a representative of the team of treating physicians to be present in the autopsy room. The physician with maximum involvement should preferably be the member of the team in the autopsy room. He should, of course, come with all the records of treatment. The knowledge of all the facets of treatment rendered before death will aid in correct interpretation of autopsy findings.

Autopsy Room Assistant. During the moments of getting ready for the autopsy, the assistant should keep all instruments, containers, dictating equipment, etc., ready. He should be instructed not to do anything with the dead body unless specifically asked by the pathologist. Removal of the organs should be done by the pathologist. Procedures such as sawing of the skull, removal of the spinal cord, etc., performed by the autopsy room assistant must be carried out under the pathologist's strict supervision.

Photographer. Needless to say the photographer picked to take the pictures in the autopsy room should be an experienced and discreet one. He should be ready with cameras that have been proven to give good photographs. One camera should be loaded with black-and-white film and another with color film for prints. He should be instructed to take photographs only when asked to do so. In order to avoid confusion no other persons should be allowed to take photographs. It is advisable to keep a movie camera with color film ready. This will be useful if certain steps of dissection are to be filmed.

Medical Secretary. Secretarial assistance from a medical secretary capable of taking shorthand will help document the findings while the autopsy is being performed. In addition to dictating the findings to a secretary, or in lieu of it, the findings may be recorded on a dictating machine. Such dictations serve the main purpose of recording all the facts while they are being observed. The dictation may be typed up later, at which time one may edit the material to correct any errors.

Liaison Officer. While the autopsy is being conducted it may be necessary to receive information from various investigators outside the autopsy room or to transmit information to them. This can best be done by a liaison officer. He can respond to telephone calls and be in charge of security of the autopsy room. He can also handle inquiries from the news media.

This list should, of course, be varied depending on the circumstances of the case. It may not be necessary to have, for instance, a representative from the team of physicians administering treatment before death if consultations have been held with him prior to autopsy. One of the representatives from the FBI and the local police department may be able to undertake additional tasks of taking photographs or acting as security or liaison officer. On the other hand, it may be necessary to add to the team other aides such as radiologist, an x-ray technician or a medical illustrator. If the deceased is a foreign national, a representative of the embassy may be invited. In order to avoid confusion, it is advisable to keep to a minimum the number of people in the autopsy room and to define beforehand the role of each individual included in the team. If any questions remain unanswered, there should be no hesitation in summoning additional consultants. For legal technicalities, the responsible state's prosecuting attorney or U.S. district attorney should be consulted.

THE AUTOPSY

The autopsy on the body of a national figure must be complete in every sense of the word. This is because questions least expected are likely to be raised at the time of autopsy and many months or years later. A complete autopsy should include, among other things, consideration of the circumstances of shooting, study of medical treatment from injury to death and correlation of these facts with the findings of the autopsy. The external examination must be detailed and all questions related to the distance of fire, angle of fire, type of firearm and ammunition, etc., must be considered before the external injuries are cut out or altered in any way. Internal examination should include careful exploration of missile tracks, assessment of damage and disease, and evaluation of complications of injuries.

Collection of specimens for additional examinations is an important aspect of an autopsy. In a case of national importance, one never knows what questions will be raised. Therefore, it is advisable to keep more materials than might be considered necessary at a more routine autopsy. It could be very embarrassing to come up short at a later date.

The clothes must be retained. All extraneous material on the clothes and on the body must be carefully picked up and placed in properly identified containers. Samples of hair should be retained for these may be needed for comparison. Blood, bile and urine should be withdrawn and portions of the liver, kidneys, brain and lung kept. The blood may be needed for determining the blood groups and the other materials may be needed for toxicological analyses.

Portions of all normal and abnormal tissues must be retained for examination; representative sections of various organs including portions of the gastrointestinal tract, skeletal muscle, skin, lymph nodes and bone marrow should be kept for microscopic examination. Areas of skin bearing gunshot wounds should be retained for histological and other examinations.

There may be considerable pressure from many sources for a quick release of the body. The autopsy should be performed as rapidly as is consistent with only the best examination. Nothing should be left undone, and the investigation should not be hurried through because of demands for early release of the body. Requests for only a partial autopsy should be courteously but firmly declined.

After the autopsy is completed, the team must go over the entire course of autopsy to determine if anything has been left undone. Only after such consideration should the body be released.

RESPONSE TO QUESTIONS FROM NEWS MEDIA

The investigators will be faced with questions from the news media at all stages of the investigation. The questions will have to be answered responsibly and as fully as possible. The most important consideration in answering the questions must be, of course, that the answers should in no way affect the outcome of the judicial process to follow.

At the beginning of the investigation and autopsy, a statement should be prepared for the news media. This statement should include a brief outline of what is going to be done, the time and place of autopsy and the names of the organizations to be involved in the investigation.

Approximate time of completion of the autopsy and the approximate time and place of the next statement may be stated. No questions should be entertained at this time.

After the autopsy is completed, the pathologist in charge of the autopsy together with other investigators may hold a news conference. The attorney in legal charge of the case should be consulted before such conference. In the initial statement at the news conference and during the period of questioning, it is appropriate to give the details of the procedural aspects of the investigation, state the cause of death and reveal factual data from the autopsy about which no questions of interpretation exist. Everyone on the panel must avoid getting involved in answering questions that call for opinions on theories, rumors and unfinished investigations.

THE AUTOPSY REPORT

The autopsy report must include all relevant information related to autopsy studies. The place and date of autopsy, times of commencement and completion of autopsy and the names and designations of all persons involved in the autopsy and all other persons consulted at various stages of investigation should be included in the report. The body of the report should include the following:

1. A brief statement about the circumstances of shooting and details of examination of the scene of shooting
2. Details of treatment rendered prior to death
3. Description of the clothing and extraneous materials on the body
4. Details of external and internal examinations, and microscopic examinations of skin wounds and internal organs
5. Reports of x-rays taken before and after death
6. Representative photographs with detailed legends
7. Reports of toxicological analyses, blood typing, test firings and other studies
8. Clinicopathologic correlation of autopsy findings with a summary of the case
9. A statement about the cause of death with signatures of the pathologists

THREE AUTOPSIES COMPARED

THE AUTOPSY ON THE BODY OF PRESIDENT ABRAHAM LINCOLN

On April 14, 1865, President Lincoln was shot in the back of his head with a brass-barreled derringer when he was watching a performance in Ford's Theatre in Washington, D.C. Initial treatment consisted of pouring of brandy and water in the President's mouth and removal of an obstructing clot of blood from the head wound to relieve pressure on the brain. One of the physicians treating the President was the Surgeon General of the United States. Efforts to localize the bullet were made by introducing first a Nélaton probe, then a doctor's finger, then an ordinary silver probe and finally a longer Nélaton probe. The ball could be felt by this last effort but could not be removed. The President died nine hours and seven minutes after being shot.

An autopsy was performed by Assistant Surgeon Woodward five hours after death in the President's bedroom at the White House. His report follows.[5]

Autopsy Report: President Abraham Lincoln

Surgeon General's Office
Washington City, D.C.
April 15th, 1865
Brigadier General J. K. Barnes
Surgeon General U.S.A.

General:

I have the honor to report that in obedience to your orders and aided by Assistant Surgeon E. Curtis, U.S.A., I made in your presence at 12 o'clock this morning an autopsy on the body of President Abraham Lincoln, with the following results. The eyelids and surrounding parts of the face were greatly echymosed and the eyes somewhat protuberant from effusion of blood into the orbits.

There was a gunshot wound of the head around which the scalp was greatly thickened by hemorrhage into its tissues. The ball entered through the occipital bone about one inch to the left of the median line and just above the left lateral sinus, which it opened. It then penetrated the dura mater, passed through the left posterior lobe of the cerebrum, entered the left lateral ventrical and lodged in the white matter of the cerebrum just above the anterior portion of the left corpus striatum, where it was found.

The wound in the occipital bone was quite smooth, circular in shape, with bevelled edges. The opening through the internal table being larger than that through the external table. The track of the ball was full of clotted blood and contained several little fragments of bone with a small piece of the ball near its external orifice. The brain around the track was pultaceous and livid from capillary hemorrhage into its substance. The ventricles of the brain were full of clotted blood. A thick clot beneath the dura mater coated the right cerebral lobe.

There was a smaller clot under the dura mater of the left side. But little blood was found at the base of the brain. Both the orbital plates of the frontal bone were fractured and the fragments pushed upwards towards the brain. The dura mater over these fractures were uninjured. The orbits were gorged with blood. I have the honor of being very respectfully your obedient servant.

E. J. J. Woodward
Assistant Surgeon
U.S.A.

CRITIQUE OF AUTOPSY ON THE BODY OF PRESIDENT JOHN F. KENNEDY

After the assassination of President John F. Kennedy, President Johnson appointed a commission, known as the Warren Commission, to investigate the assassination and prepare a report. Despite an extensive investigation by the President's Commission, many questions are still being raised about the circumstances of the shooting. In general, there are two main lines of thought. One body of opinion believes, as did the President's Commission, that President Kennedy was assassinated by a single assassin.[3,4,7] On the other hand, some investigators feel that more than one gun was involved.[8] A more thorough medicolegal investigation might have provided answers to at least some of the questions now being raised.

It is always easy to criticize after the fact. However, serious errors of omission and commission were made in the medicolegal investigation of the fatal shooting of President Kennedy, and they must be pointed out. In an important case such as this one, it should be possible to do everything necessary so as not to leave room for criticism.

Authority to Perform Autopsy.   President Kennedy was pronounced dead at Parkland Hospital, Dallas, Texas. Legally the Texas authorities had the right and duty to perform the autopsy in Texas. A competent pathologist with extensive experience in Forensic Pathology who was the Medical Examiner in Dallas should have been allowed to conduct the autopsy with the help of other pathologists. The military authorities should not have forced the removal of the President's body to the U.S. Naval Hospital in Bethesda, Maryland. They did not have legal authority to force the removal of the body out of Texas. *AFTER ALL, THOUGH, IS A*

Selection of Pathologists.   An autopsy on the body of a national figure, as has been pointed out, must be performed with great care by persons experienced in Forensic Pathology. Even in straightforward situations, many questions will be raised based on rumors and conflicting stories. Without a thorough and reliable investigation in the autopsy room, it may not be possible to answer these questions satisfactorily. In the case of President Kennedy, the authorities assuming charge of the autopsy investigations asked military pathologists who had only limited experience in performing autopsies on medicolegal cases to proceed with the autopsy. Even with such circumstances as existed at the time, it would have been possible to summon experienced civilian forensic pathologists to perform the autopsy without causing any undue delay.

Pre-Autopsy Investigation.   The pathologists proceeded to examine and interpret the wounds on the President's body without bothering to find out what had been done in the hospital to revive the President.

This failure in following the basic principle of medicolegal investigation initially led to serious misinterpretation of the gunshot wound on the front of the President's neck.

Autopsy Room Environment. It is apparent that there was considerable confusion in the autopsy room during the course of autopsy. Far too many people, numbering at least thirty, were present in the autopsy room at one time or another.[8] Wecht and Smith have noted the occurrence of a disturbing episode of seizure of a roll of film exposed by a medical corpsman during the autopsy and its destruction by a Secret Service agent.[8] It is also alleged that an Army General exerted excessive influence on the pathologists and made them rush through the investigation. For one reason or another, the pathologists did not make a complete postmortem examination. For instance, they did not dissect the wound in the upper part of the back and did not explore the track of the wound. The brain, which was left for fixation, was not examined completely; the autopsy report states that "In the interest of preserving the specimen coronal sections were not made."

Autopsy Report. Several deficiencies are obvious in the autopsy report, which is reproduced below in its entirety. First, the report is not dated and the time of completion of autopsy is not stated. Secondly, the descriptions of the gunshot wounds are incomplete: the measurements from the top of the head and from midline to the wounds (which can determine the precise location of wounds) are not included in the report, and no mention of the reconstruction of the wounds and of evaluation of the bullet tracks is made. Thirdly, the weights and descriptions of all of the abdominal organs are missing from the report. Fourthly, even though President Kennedy was believed to have Addison's disease, the gross and microscopic descriptions of the adrenal glands have not been included in the report. Finally, no description of the President's clothes is included in the autopsy report, and the information about the correlation of bullet holes in the clothing and the gunshot wounds on the body is missing.

Interpretation of the Autopsy Findings. Incomplete autopsy has been a factor, at least in part, in the lingering of doubts about whether the President was shot with one gun or two. Major controversy surrounds the interpretation of the angle of fire. The Warren Commission diagrams indicate that the angle made by the bullet track in the President's neck with the horizontal was about 10 degrees (Fig. 16-1).[7] Independent researchers who have studied the autopsy photographs, x-rays and other materials feel that the angle was more than 20 degrees (Fig. 16-2).[4,8] There are also differences in the diagrams of the head wounds prepared by the Warren Commission and by private investigators (Figs. 16-3, 16-4)[4,7]

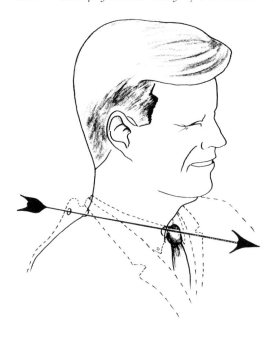

Fig. 16-1. The neck wound, based on the Warren Commission report.

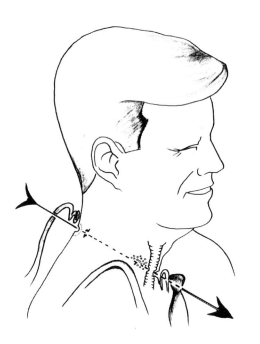

Fig. 16-2. A diagram, based on the interpretations of independent researchers, showing a greater angle of the bullet track with the horizontal.

Fig. 16-3. A diagram, based on the Warren Commission report, showing the head wound.

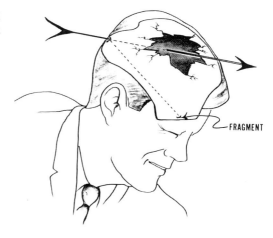

FRAGMENT

Fig. 16-4. A diagram, based on the interpretations by independent researchers, showing more details and different angle of the bullet track.

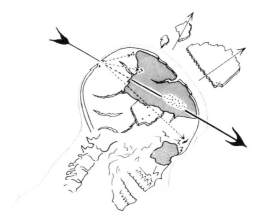

Autopsy Report: President John F. Kennedy

Date and Hour Died: 22 November 1963 1300 (CST).

Date and Hour Autopsy Performed: 22 November 1963 2000 (EST).

Prosector: (497831) Cdr. J. J. Humes, MC, USN; Assistant: (489878) Cdr. "J" Thornton Boswell, MC, USN; LCol. Pierre A. Finck, MC, USA (04 043 322).

Clinical diagnoses (Including Operations): Ht.—72½ inches; Wt.—170 pounds; Eyes—blue; Hair—Reddish brown.

Pathological Diagnoses: CAUSE OF DEATH; gunshot wound, head.

Approved—Signature: J. J. Humes, Cdr. MC, USN.

Military Organization: President, United States.

Age 46; Sex: male; Race: Cauc.; Autopsy No.: A63-272.

Patient's Identification: Kennedy, John F.; Naval Medical School.

Clinical Summary: According to available information the deceased, President John F. Kennedy, was riding in an open car in a motorcade during an official visit to Dallas, Texas, on 22 November 1963. The President was sitting in the right rear seat with Mrs. Kennedy seated on the same seat to his left. Sitting directly in front of the President was Governor John B. Connally of Texas and directly in front of Mrs. Kennedy sat Mrs. Connally. The vehicle was moving at a slow rate of speed down an incline into an underpass that leads to a freeway route to the Dallas Trade Mart where the President was to deliver an address.

Three shots were heard and the President fell forward bleeding from the head. (Governor Connally was seriously wounded by the same gunfire.) According to newspaper reports (Washington Post, November 22, 1963) Bob Jackson, a Dallas Times Herald Photographer, said he looked around as he heard the shots and saw a rifle barrel disappearing into a window on the upper floor of the nearby Texas School Book Depository Building.

Shortly following the wounding of the two men the car was driven to Parkland Hospital in Dallas. In the emergency room of that hospital the President was attended by Dr. Malcolm Perry. Telephone communication with Dr. Perry on November 23, 1963, develops the following information relative to the observations made by Dr. Perry and procedures performed there prior to death.

Dr. Perry noted the massive wound of the head and a second much smaller wound of the low anterior neck in approximately the midline. A tracheostomy was performed by extending the latter wound. At this point bloody air was noted bubbling from the wound and injury to the right lateral wall of the trachea was observed. Incisions were made in the upper anterior chest wall bilaterally to combat possible subcutaneous emphysema. Intravenous infusions of blood and saline were begun and oxygen was administered. Despite these measures cardiac arrest occurred and closed chest cardiac massage failed to re-establish cardiac action. The President was pronounced dead approximately thirty to forty minutes after receiving his wounds.

The remains were transported via the presidential plane to Washington, D.C., and subsequently to the Naval Medical School, National Naval Medical Center, Bethesda, Maryland for postmortem examination.

GENERAL DESCRIPTION OF BODY: The body is that of a muscular, well-developed and well-nourished adult Caucasian male measuring 72½ inches and weighing approximately 170 pounds. There is beginning rigor mortis, minimal dependent livor mortis of the dorsum, and early algor mortis. The hair is reddish brown and abundant, the eyes are blue, the right pupil measuring 8 mm in diameter, the left 4 mm. There is edema and ecchymosis of the inner canthus region of the left eyelid measuring approximately 1.5 cm in greatest diameter. There is edema and ecchymosis diffusely over the right supra-orbital ridge with abnormal mobility of the underlying bone. (The remainder of the scalp will be described with the skull.) There is clotted blood on the external ears but otherwise the ears, nares, and mouth are essentially unremarkable. The teeth are in excellent repair and there is some pallor of the oral mucous membrane.

Situated on the upper right posterior thorax just above the upper border of the scapula there is a 7 × 4 mm oval wound. This wound is measured to be 14 cm from the tip of the right acromion process and 14 cm below the tip of the right mastoid process.

Situated in the low anterior neck at approximately the level of the third and fourth tracheal rings is a 6.5 cm long transverse wound with widely gaping irregular edges. (The depth and character of these wounds will be further described below.)

Situated on the anterior chest wall in the nipple line are bilateral 2 cm long recent transverse surgical incisions into the subcutaneous tissue. The one on the left is situated 11 cm cephalad to the nipple and the one on the right 8 cm cephalad to the nipple. There is no hemorrhage or ecchymosis associated with these wounds. A similar clear wound measuring 2 cm in length is situated on the anterolateral aspect of the left midarm. Situated on the anterolateral aspect of each ankle is a recent 2 cm transverse incision into the subcutaneous tissue.

There is an old well-healed 8 cm McBurney abdominal incision. Over the lumbar spine in the midline is an old, well-healed 15 cm scar. Situated on the upper anterolateral aspect of the right thigh is an old, well-healed 8 cm scar.

MISSILE WOUNDS: 1. There is a large irregular defect of the scalp and skull on the right involving chiefly the parietal bone but extending somewhat into the temporal and occipital regions. In this region there is an actual absence of scalp and bone producing a defect which measures approximately 13 cm in greatest diameter.

From the irregular margins of the above scalp defect tears extend in stellate fashion into the more or less intact scalp as follows:

a. From the right inferior temporo-parietal margin anterior to the right ear to a point slightly above the tragus.

b. From the anterior parietal margin anteriorly on the forehead to approximately 4 cm above the right orbital ridge.

c. From the left margin of the main defect across the midline anterolaterally for a distance of approximately 8 cm.

d. From the same starting point as c. 10 cm posterolaterally. Situated in the posterior scalp approximately 2.5 cm laterally to the right and slightly above the external occipital protuberance is a lacerated wound measuring 15 × 6 mm. In the underlying bone is a corresponding wound through the skull which exhibits beveling of the margins of the bone when viewed from the inner aspect of the skull.

Clearly visible in the above described large skull defect and exuding from it is lacerated brain tissue which on close inspection proves to represent the major portion of the right cerebral hemisphere. At this point it is noted that the falx cerebri is extensively lacerated with disruption of the superior saggital sinus.

Upon reflecting the scalp multiple complete fracture lines are seen to radiate from both the large defect at the vertex and the smaller wound at the occiput. These vary greatly in length and direction, the longest measuring approximately 19 cm. These result in the production of numerous fragments which vary in size from a few millimeters to 10 cm in greatest diameter.

The complexity of these fractures and the fragments thus produced tax satisfactory verbal description and are better appreciated in photographs and roentgenograms which are prepared.

The brain is removed and preserved for further study following formalin fixation.

Received as separate specimens from Dallas, Texas are three fragments of skull bone which in aggregate roughly approximate the dimensions of the large defect described above. At one angle of the largest of these fragments is a portion of the perimeter of a roughly circular wound presumably of exit which exhibits beveling of the outer aspect of the bone and is estimated to measure approximately 2.5 to 3.0 cm in diameter. Roentgenograms of this fragment reveal minute particles of metal in the bone at this margin. Roentgenograms of the skull reveal multiple minute metallic fragments along a line corresponding with a line joining the above described small occipital wound and the right supraorbital ridge. From the surface of the disrupted right cerebral cortex two small irregularly shaped fragments of metal are recovered. These measure 7 × 2 mm and 3 × 1 mm. These are placed in the custody of Agents Francis X. O'Neill, Jr., and James W. Sibert, of the Federal Bureau of Investigation, who executed a receipt therefor (attached).

2. The second wound presumably of entry is that described above in the upper right posterior thorax. Beneath the skin there is ecchymosis of subcutaneous tissue and musculature. The missile path through the fascia and musculature cannot be easily probed. The wound presumably of exit was that described by Dr. Malcolm Perry of Dallas in the low anterior cervical region. When observed by Dr. Perry the wound measured "a few millimeters in diameter"; however it was extended as a tracheostomy incision and thus its character is distorted at the time of autopsy. However, there is considerable ecchymosis of the strap muscles of the right side of the neck and of the fascia about the trachea adjacent to the line of the tracheostomy wound. The third point of reference in connecting these two wounds is in the apex (supraclavicular portion) of the right pleural cavity. In this region there is contusion of the parietal pleura and of the extreme apical portion of the right upper lobe of the lung. In both instances the diameter of contusion and ecchymosis at the point of maximal involvement measures 5 cm. Both the visceral and parietal pleura are intact overlying these areas of trauma.

INCISIONS: The scalp wounds are extended in the coronal plane to examine the cranial content and the customary (Y) shaped incision is used to examine the body cavities.

THORACIC CAVITY: The bony cage is unremarkable. The thoracic organs are in their normal positions and relationships and there is no increase in free pleural fluid. The above described area of contusion in the apical portion of the right pleural cavity is noted.

LUNGS: The lungs are of essentially similar appearance, the right weighing 320 g, the left 290 g. The lungs are well aerated with smooth glistening pleural surfaces and gray-pink color. A 5-cm-diameter area of purplish red discoloration and increased firmness to palpation is situated in the apical portion of the right upper lobe. This corresponds to the similar area described in the overlying parietal pleura. Incision in this region reveals recent hemorrhage into pulmonary parenchyma.

HEART: The pericardial cavity is smooth walled and contains approximately 10 cc of straw-colored fluid. The heart is of essentially normal external contour and weighs 350 g. The pulmonary artery is opened in situ and no abnormalities are noted. The cardiac chambers contain moderate amounts of postmortem clotted blood. There are no gross abnormalities of the leaflets of any of the cardiac valves. The following are the circumferences of the cardiac valves: aortic 7.5 cm, pulmonic 7 cm, tricuspid 12 cm, mitral 11 cm. The myocardium is firm and reddish brown. The left ventricular myocardium averages 1.2 cm in thickness, the right ventricular myocardium 0.4 cm. The coronary arteries are dissected and are of normal distribution and smooth-walled and elastic throughout.

ABDOMINAL CAVITY: The abdominal organs are in their normal positions and relationships and there is no increase in free peritoneal fluid. The vermiform appendix is surgically absent and there are a few adhesions joining the region of the cecum to the ventral abdominal wall at the above described old abdominal incisional scar.

SKELETAL SYSTEM: Aside from the above described skull wounds there are no significant gross skeletal abnormalities.

PHOTOGRAPHY: Black-and-white and color photographs depicting significant findings are exposed but not developed. These photographs were placed in the custody of Agent Roy H. Kellerman of the U.S. Secret Service, who executed a receipt therefor (attached).

ROENTGENOGRAMS: Roentgenograms are made of the entire body and of the separately submitted three fragments of skull bone. These are developed and were placed in the custody of Agent Roy H. Kellerman of the U.S. Secret Service, who executed a receipt therefor (attached).

SUMMARY: Based on the above observations it is our opinion that the deceased died as a result of two perforating gunshot wounds inflicted by high velocity projectiles fired by a person or persons unknown. The projectiles were fired from a point behind and somewhat above the level of the deceased. The observations and available information do not permit a satisfactory estimate as to the sequence of the two wounds.

The fatal missile entered the skull above and to the right of the external occipital protuberance. A portion of the projectile traversed the cranial cavity in a posterior-anterior direction (see lateral skull roentgenograms), depositing minute particles along its path. A portion of the projectile made its exit through the parietal bone on the right carrying with it portions of cerebrum, skull and scalp. The two wounds of the skull combined with the force of the missile produced extensive fragmentation of the skull, lacerations of the superior saggital sinus, and of the right cerebral hemisphere.

The other missile entered the right superior posterior thorax above the scapula and traversed the soft tissues of the supra-scapular and the supra-clavicular portions of the base of the right side of the neck. This missile produced contusions of the right apical parietal pleura and of the apical portion of the right upper lobe of the lung. The missile contused the strap muscles of the right side of the neck, damaged the trachea, and made its exit through the anterior surface of the neck. As far as can be ascertained this missile struck no bony structures in its path through the body.

In addition, it is our opinion that the wound of the skull produced such extensive damage to the brain as to preclude the possibility of the deceased surviving this injury.

A supplementary report will be submitted following more detailed examination of the brain and of microscopic sections. However, it is not anticipated that these examinations will materially alter the findings.

(signed)

J. J. HUMES	"J" THORNTON BOSWELL	PIERRE A. FINCK
CDR, MC, USN (497831)	CDR, MC, USN (489878)	LT COL, MC, USA
		(04-043-322)

SUPPLEMENTARY REPORT OF AUTOPSY NUMBER A 63-272
PRESIDENT JOHN F. KENNEDY

GROSS DESCRIPTION OF BRAIN: Following formalin fixation the brain weighs 1,500 g. The right cerebral hemisphere is found to be markedly disrupted. There is a longitudinal laceration of the right hemisphere which is para-sagittal in position approximately 2.5 cm to the right of the midline which extends from the tip of the occipital lobe posteriorly to the tip of the frontal lobe anteriorly. The base of the laceration is situated approximately 4.5 cm below the vertex in the white matter. There is considerable loss of cortical substance above the base of the laceration, particularly in the parietal lobe. The margins of this laceration are at all points jagged and irregular, with additional lacerations extending in varying directions and for varying distances from the main laceration. In addition, there is a laceration of the corpus callosum extending from the genu to the tail. Exposed in this latter laceration are the interiors of the right lateral and third ventricles.

When viewed from the vertex the left cerebral hemisphere is intact. There is marked engorgement of meningeal blood vessels of the left temporal and frontal regions with considerable associated subarachnoid hemorrhage. The gyri and sulci over the left hemisphere are of essentially normal size and distribution. Those on the right are too fragmented and distorted for satisfactory description.

When viewed from the basilar aspect the disruption of the right cortex is again obvious. There is a longitudinal laceration of the mid-brain through the floor of the third ventricle just behind the optic chiasm and the mammillary bodies. This laceration partially communicates with an oblique 1.5-cm-tear through the left cerebral peduncle. There are irregular superficial lacerations over the basilar aspects of the left temporal and frontal lobes.

In the interest of preserving the specimen coronal sections are not made. The following sections are taken for microscopic examination:

a. From the margin of the laceration in the right parietal lobe.
b. From the margin of the laceration in the corpus callosum.
c. From the anterior portion of the laceration in the right frontal lobe.
d. From the contused left fronto-parietal cortex.
e. From the line of transection of the spinal cord.
f. From the right cerebellar cortex.
g. From the superficial laceration of the basilar aspect of the left temporal lobe.

During the course of this examination seven (7) black-and-white and six (6) color 4 × 5-inch negatives are exposed but not developed (the cassettes containing these negatives have been delivered by hand to Rear Admiral George W. Burkley, MC, USN, White House Physician).

MICROSCOPIC EXAMINATION:

BRAIN: Multiple sections from representative areas as noted above are examined. All sections are essentially similar and show extensive disruption of brain tissue with associated hemorrhage. In none of the sections examined are there significant abnormalities other than those directly related to the recent trauma.

HEART: Sections show a moderate amount of subepicardial fat. The coronary arteries, myocardial fibers, and endocardium are unremarkable.

LUNGS: Sections through the grossly described area of contusion in the right upper lobe exhibit disruption of alveolar walls and recent hemorrhage into alveoli. Sections are otherwise essentially unremarkable.

LIVER: Sections show the normal hepatic architecture to be well preserved. The parenchymal cells exhibit markedly granular cytoplasm indicating high glycogen content which is characteristic of the "liver biopsy pattern" of sudden death.

SPLEEN: Sections show no significant abnormalities.

KIDNEYS: Sections show no significant abnormalities aside from dilatation and engorgement of blood vessels of all calibers.

SKIN WOUNDS: Sections through the wounds in the occipital and upper right posterior thoracic regions are essentially similar. In each there is loss of continuity of the epidermis with coagulation necrosis of the tissues at the wound margins. The scalp wound exhibits several small fragments of bone at its margins in the subcutaneous tissue.

FINAL SUMMARY: This supplementary report covers in more detail the extensive degree of cerebral trauma in this case. However, neither this portion of the examination nor the microscopic examination alter the previously submitted report or add significant details to the cause of death.

J. J. HUMES
CDR, MC, USN, 497831
6 December 1963

COMMENTS ON THE
AUTOPSY ON THE BODY OF SENATOR ROBERT F. KENNEDY

The report of autopsy on the body of Senator Kennedy is a classic document and should serve as an example to follow when dealing with the investigation of a tragedy of national importance.

The entire investigation was carried out smoothly. The line of jurisdiction was clearly established, and the Chief Medical Examiner—Coroner of Los Angeles County, Dr. Thomas T. Noguchi, who had the legal authority to conduct the autopsy—was clearly in charge of the investigation. He selected an adequately equipped place for autopsy investigation and rightly placed a man in charge of security of the autopsy room. He sought advice from various consultants. A radiologist and members of the neurosurgical team that treated the Senator were present at the autopsy. Two forensic pathologists assisted in the autopsy and three other pathologists, including a neuropathologist, were invited to serve as consultants. Three forensic and medical photographers took pictures, and one aide was in charge of interagency relations. Advice was sought after the autopsy from several forensic pathologists.

The autopsy itself, which lasted 6¼ hours, was followed by further investigations such as the examinations of the scene, test firings and special photographic and radiographic studies. A general toxicological analysis of blood, liver and lungs was made and ABO and Rh typing of the blood performed. The microscopic examination of various body tissues was exhaustive.

The autopsy report gives all relevant details of clothing, findings of external and internal examinations, results of various post-autopsy investigations mentioned above, together with the chronology of events of investigations and the personnel involved.[6] Parts of this autopsy protocol, dealing with the examination of clothing, general external examination, examination of gunshot wounds and brain, and the final summary are reproduced here.

Autopsy Report: Senator Robert F. Kennedy

EXAMINATION OF CLOTHING AT THE TIME OF AUTOPSY

1. There is a dark blue, fine worsted-type suit coat bearing the label "Georgetown University Shop-Georgetown, D.C." The coat has been cut

and/or torn at the left yoke and left sleeve area. The right sleeve is intact There is variable blood staining over the right shoulder region and on the right lapel. Two apparent bullet holes are identified in the right axillary region, slightly over 1 inch (2.5 cm) and slightly over 1¼ inch (3.2 cm) from the underseam area, respectively, and corresponding with wounds described on the body elsewhere in this report. Also noted at the top of the right shoulder region centered about 1¼ inches from the shoulder seam and about ⅝ inch (1.6 cm) posterior to the yoke seam superiorly is an irregular rent of the fabric, somewhat less than 1¼ inch (3.2 cm) in diameter and definitely everting superficially and upward. The three front buttons of the garment are intact. (Subsequent examination of the coat showed the presence of a superficial through-and-through bullet path through the upper right shoulder area, passing through the suit fabric proper but not the lining.)

2. There is a pair of trousers of matching material with a very dark leather belt with rectangular metal buckle and showing the gold-stamped label "Custom Leather, Reversible, 32." The zipper is intact. There is a minimal amount of apparent blood staining over the anterior portions of the trouser legs.

3. There is a white cotton shirt with the label "K WRAGGE, 48 West 46th Street, New York." The laundry mark initials "RFK" are present on the neck band. The left portion of the shirt has been disrupted in approximately the same manner as the suit coat and is similarly absent. The right cuff is intact and is of semi-French design. A chain-connected yellow metal cufflink with plain oval design is in place. A corresponding left cufflink is not among the items submitted. Apparent bullet holes are identified as corresponding to those in the previously described area of suit coat.

4. There is a tie of apparent silk rep, navy blue with an approximately 3/16 inch (0.5 cm) gray diagonal stripe. The label is "Chase and Collier, McLean, Virginia." The marker is RIVETZ.

5. There is a pair of navy blue, nearly calf-length socks of mixed cashmere and apparently nylon fiber, the fiber content stencil labeling still being nearly discernible on the foot portions.

6. There is a pair of white broadcloth boxer-type shorts with two labels: "Sun-sheen Broadcloth V' Cloth-34"; and "Custom fashioned for Lewis and Thos. Saltz, Washington." There is a small amount of blood stain at the anterior crotch, along with pale straw-colored discoloration to the left of the fly. A few patches of dry blood are present on the back as well.

7. There is a trapezoidally folded cotton handkerchief showing, on what appears to be the presenting (anterior) surface, several scattered dark red and somewhat brown spots ranging from a fraction of a millimeter to about 4 mm (less than 3/16 inch) in greatest dimension.

8. No shoes are submitted for examination.

The above listed items are saved for further and more detailed study by others.

GENERAL EXTERNAL EXAMINATION

The nonembalmed body, measuring 70½ inches (179 cm) in length and weighing about 165 pounds (74.5 kg), is that of a well developed, well-nourished, and muscular Caucasian male appearing about the recorded age of 42 years. The extremities are generally symmetrical bilaterally, showing no obvious structural abnormality.

The head shows extensive bandaging, somewhat blood-stained in the posterior aspect. Dressings are also present in the right clavicular region, the right axilla, and the right ankle regions. Also present over the right inguinofemoral region are apparently elastoplast dressings. A recent tracheostomy has been performed at a comparatively low level. A clear plastic tracheostomy tube fitted with an inflatable cuff is in place. The area also shows a gauze dressing. Lividity is well developed in the posterior aspect of the body, mainly at the upper shoulder and midback regions with approximately equal distribution bilaterally. The lividity blanches definitely on finger pressure.

Rigor mortis is not detected in the extremities or in the neck. (Rigor was noted to be developing in the arms and legs by the time of conclusion of the autopsy.)

A complete examination of the external surfaces of the body is undertaken following removal of all dressings.

The head contour is generally symmetrical, due allowance being made for the soft-tissue edema and hemorrhage in the right postauricular region in general. The hair is graying light brown and of male distribution. Portions of the right half of the scalp have been clipped and/or shaved. Hair in the inguinal and femoral regions has also been shaved in part. Hair texture is medium.

There is an irregularly bordered area of comparatively recent yet pale ecchymosis centered about 1 inch (2.5 cm) above the midportion of the right eyebrow. Marked ecchymosis with moderate edema is present in the right periorbital region but mainly of the upper eyelid. No hemorrhage or generalized congestion is seen in the conjunctival or scleral membranes. The nose is symmetrical, showing no evidence of fracture or hemorrhage. The glabella shows no evidence of trauma. Eye color is hazel. Pupillary diameters are equal at about 5 mm (3/16 inch).

The buccal mucosa and the tongue show no lesion.

Chest diameters are within normal limits and there is bilateral symmetry. The breasts are those of a normal adult male. The abdomen is scaphoid. No abdominal scar is identified. There is an old low medial inguinal scar on the right.

Texture and configuration of the nails are within normal limits, and no focal lesions are noted. There is no peripheral edema.

The skin in general shows a smooth texture and no additional significant focal lesion. There is abundant suntan, especially at the neck region where its contrast with the areas shaved for surgical preparation on the right can be noted.

No structural abnormality is noted on the back.

There is a diagonally disposed recent surgical incision about 3 inches (7.5 cm) in length in the right anterolateral femoral region. This incision has been intactly sutured. There is an associated plastic tubing of small diameter, centered about 1/2 inch (12 mm) from the infero-medial margin of the incision.

Also noted in a comparable location on the left are several hypodermic puncture marks. These just mentioned areas show the presence of red-orange dye.

There are recent cutdowns at the right ankle and the lateral right knee with thin polyethylene tubes in place. No extravasation is noted.

The external genitalia are those of a normal circumcised adult male.

DESCRIPTION OF GUNSHOT WOUNDS

Gunshot Wound No. 1

The wound of entry, as designated by Maxwell M. Andler, Jr., M.D., neurosurgeon attending the autopsy, and more or less evident by inspection of the apposed craniotomy incision, is centered 5 inches (12.7 cm) from the vertex, about ¾ inch (1.9 cm) posterior to the center of the right external auditory meatus, about ¾ inch (1.9 cm) superior to the Reid line, and 2½ inches (6.4 cm) anterior to a coronal plane passing through the occipital protuberance at its scalp-covered aspect. The defect appears to have been about 3/16 inch (0.5 cm) in diameter at the skin surface. The surgical incision passing through the area of the wound of entry has been fashioned in a semilunar configuration with the concavity directed inferiorly and posteriorly. The incision has been intactly sutured by metallic and other material. The arc length is about 4 inches (10 cm). Further detailed description of the area is given elsewhere in this report.

Varyingly moderate degrees of very recent hemorrhage are noted in the soft tissue inferior to the right mastoid region, extending medially as well. There is no hematoma in the soft tissue. In conjunction with the wound of entry, the right external ear shows, on the posterior aspect of the helix, an irregularly fusiform zone of dark red and gray stippling about one inch (2.5 cm) in greatest dimension, along the posterior cartilaginous border and over a maximum width of about ¼ inch (0.5 cm) at the midportion of the stippled zone. This widest zone of stippling is approximately along a radius originating from the wound of entry in the right mastoid region. Moderate edema and variable ecchymosis is present in the associated portions of right external ear as well.

No evidence of powder burn, tattoo, or stippling is found in the area surrounding the wound of entry of Gunshot Wound No. 1, to include an arbitrary circular zone superimposed upon the above-described stippling on the right ear.

LESIONS IN DETAIL (NEUROPATHOLOGY)

A. Scalp and Cranium

A U-shaped recent surgical wound is present over the right temporo-occipital region of the recently shaved scalp behind the right ear. Many wire sutures are in place. About 2 cm above the tip of the mastoid process immediately behind the pinna at about the level of the external auditory meatus, the anterior portion of the skin of the incision shows a semicircular defect said to be a portion of the original bullet entrance wound (according to the surgeons who were present at the examination). After removing the wire sutures, the scalp is incised by the usual mastoid-to-mastoid incision across the vertex. The incision on the right is extended into the surgical incision mentioned above. After reflecting the scalp, dark red subcutaneous and subgaleal hemorrhages are found in the right temporo-occipital region overlying and around the wound and the surgical craniotomy over an area measuring 9.5 × 10 cm. The hemorrhage ranges up to 3 mm in thickness. The right temporal muscle shows a small amount of hemorrhage along its posterior aspect.

The bony defect of the cranium included the superior portions of the right mastoid process and the adjacent temporo-occipital bones in an irregularly oval area measuring 6 × 5 cm. Gelfoam and hemorrhagic material is removed from the craniotomy site. A circumferential cut with three notches is made in the calvarium with a vibratory saw. The calvarium is removed from the underlying dura. There is no lesion in this portion of the cranium.

The bone surrounding the craniotomy is removed in a single piece, including the posterior half of the right external auditory canal. The bullet wound in the skull appears to be located with its anterior margin 1 cm posterior to the right external auditory meatus, 2 cm superior to the tip of the mastoid process; but the original configuration is obscured by the surgical enlargement and by the adjacent craniotomy. The surgical opening of the right temporo-occipital bone measures 6 cm anteroposteriorly and 5 cm supero-inferiorly. Burr holes, saw cuts, and rongeur cuts can be seen along the margins of the bone.

The bullet wound of the mastoid extends medially to the base of the petrous portion where there is a triangular defect with the base of the triangle corresponding to the petrous ridge and measuring 8 mm in width.

A curved fracture about 1 cm long is found in the central thinnest portion of the right supra-orbital plate with intra-orbital hemorrhage beneath it surrounding the right eye. A laceration of the dura and contusion of the right orbital gyri are located above the fracture.

B. Meninges, blood vessels, and cranial nerves

In the dorsolateral aspect of the subdural space there is a film of blood up to 3 mm thick, covering the arachnoid over both posterior frontal and parieto-occipital regions and extending downward to, and in some places below the sylvian fissure bilaterally, slightly more on the left side than on the right. Similar blood clot is also found on the left middle fossa and in both posterior fossae, again more on the left side. A small amount of blood clot, about 2 cc, is found between the cerebral hemispheres just dorsal to the midbrain.

Rather diffuse subarachnoid hemorrhage is present over the parieto-occipital regions, over the dorsal and right side of the cerebellum, and also over the ventral surface of the pons and medulla. All of this, however, is quite slight, and the blood clot does not obscure the underlying structures.

Epidural hemorrhages are found in the following three locations:

1. Adjacent to the craniotomy defect of the right temporo-occipital region. This is minimal and extends not more than 1 cm from the surgical incision and it is less than 1 mm in thickness.
2. Above the right supraorbital plate where the fracture is present as described above. This is deemed minimal and less than 1 mm in thickness covering an area 1.5 × 1 cm.
3. Epidural hemorrhage measuring 2 cm longitudinally and 1 cm transversely is found in the dorsal aspect of the epidural space at C1 and C2 vertebral levels.

The dorsal veins which empty into the superior saggital sinus are inspected but they reveal no evidence of the source of subdural hemorrhage.

The right superior petrosal sinus is severed for a distance of 8 mm corresponding to the defect of the petrous ridge mentioned above. The remainder of this sinus adjacent to the defect has been cauterized. The tentorium which has its attachment to the right petrous ridge is lacerated where the bony defect is present. This laceration of the dura is continued laterally and communicates with the surgical defect which measures 4.5 × 2.0 cm just anterior to the right sigmoid sinus and above the transverse sinus beneath the craniotomy opening. A second surgical defect is present on the dura posterior to the sigmoid sinus and inferior to the transverse sinus and this measures 3 × 2 cm. There are areas of brownish discoloration and a minimal amount of blood clot is scattered along the margins of these dural openings.

The lateral portion of the transverse sinus and the sigmoid sinus thus transverse the craniotomy defect horizontally through its posterior portion and vertically through its inferior portion. The tentorium cerebelli shows no defects in its central portions. The dura was lacerated over a small area over the right supraorbital plate where a curved fracture was present as mentioned above.

The superior saggital sinus, left transverse sinus, left sigmoid sinus and cavernous sinuses are inspected and reveal no evidence of thrombosis or laceration. The right transverse and sigmoid sinuses do not appear to be damaged in spite of their proximity to the dural openings anterior and posterior to it, but cautery marks are on and close to these sinuses, which contain dark red blood clots.

Examination of the arteries of the brain stem and cerebellum reveals a right vertebral artery that is smaller than the left. The basilar artery measures 3 mm in diameter and is slightly tortuous. The anterior inferior cerebellar arteries and the posterior inferior cerebellar arteries have a normal distribution and show no evidence of traumatic injury. The left superior cerebellar artery is intact. The right superior cerebellar artery is intact throughout its main trunk, but several of its superficial branches are involved in the cortical contusion and laceration of the cerebellum and many of its deeper branches have been damaged by the penetrating bullet and bone fragments. All of the remaining blood vessels of the brain stem, cerebellum and cerebral hemispheres have normal distribution and show very slight atherosclerosis. There is no evidence of injury except for the areas of contusions and lacerations.

The cranial nerves are all intact.

C. Cerebrum

Slight depression of the cerebral cortex is noted over both posterior frontal and parietal convexities in the areas beneath the subdural hemorrhage that is described above. The right cerebral hemisphere is slightly larger than the left with shallow tentorium grooves over both unci, slightly more prominent on the right than on the left. However, there is no evidence of herniation of the cingulate gyri beneath the falx. The gyri over both cerebral convexities are flattened.

When the brain is inspected from the ventral aspect, three areas of contusion-laceration can be seen in the cortex of the right cerebral hemisphere and a fourth area of contusion on the left. The largest one measures 4 × 3 cm. It consists of superficial and deep lacerations and contusions of the mesial half of the posterior one-third of the right inferior temporal gyrus for an anteroposterior distance of 4 cm; the middle third of the right fusiform gyrus for 3 cm and the lateral portion of the hippocampal gyrus for a distance of about 1 cm. Coronal sections show that this laceration has a subcortical hemorrhage extending 1.5 cm into the subcortical white matter to the floor of the posterior part of the temporal horn of the right lateral ventricle with rupture into this cavity. The medial portions of the temporal lesion are characteristic of laceration and contusion, while the lateral portions of this lesion are quite characteristic of hemorrhagic infarction.

The second largest contusion is in the middle part of the right orbital gyri and measures 1.5 × 1.0 cm with a 5 mm curved laceration within it. Hemorrhage extends into the subcortical white matter to a depth of 6 mm. This lesion overlies the lacerated dura and fracture of the right supraorbital plate.

The third contusion measures 14 × 7 mm with a linear 6 mm transverse laceration and is situated in the mesial portion of the inferior part of the right occipital cortex.

The fourth contusion of the cortex is a very small lesion in the middle of the left inferior temporal gyrus and measures 5 × 2 mm. There is no laceration in this area. This condition is limited to the gray matter.

D.   Cerebellum

In the anterior and lateral aspects of the right hemisphere of the cerebellum, there is an irregular penetrating wound. The opening measures 2 × 2 cm with irregular margins. The margins of this wound and adjacent areas are elevated to form a ring of tissue at the bony margin, 2 mm distal to the internal bone surface. This indicates herniation of the cerebellar tissue into the bony defect. On the surface of this defect and in the bone incision, there are fragments of gelfoam and soft friable blood clots.

A partially collapsed linear tract measuring 5 cm in length extends from the cerebellar cortex and subcortical white matter of the cerebellum to the vermis. The tract begins just rostral to the tegmentum of the anterior one-third of the pons, anterior to the middle cerebellar peduncle and proceeds in a superior and posterior direction. From an imaginary transverse plane between the two mastoid bones, one would estimate that this tract proceeds about 45 degrees posteriorly and medially and 30 degrees superiorly from the mastoid perforation. The tract ends in the vermis of the cerebellum where a 1 cm transverse laceration is found in the region of the primary fissure, which is approximately 3 cm posterior to the anterior cerebellar notch. At the termination of the tract, hemorrhage can be seen within the cortical laceration.

The size of the penetrating wound is difficult to determine at this time since the tract is largely filled by the swollen white matter of the cerebellum and by hemorrhage. However, probing into the tract at the entrance wound indicates that it was in the order of 2 cm in width at maximal expansion.

Upon palpation and probing in the region of the laceration in the superior vermis, a metallic fragment is found just beneath the arachnoid membrane and within an area of hemorrhage. This irregular gray metallic fragment measures 6 × 3 × 2 mm and corresponds to the largest fragment that was identified in the postoperative x-ray of a radiopaque object near the midline.

In addition to the penetrating wound and the laceration of the vermis at its terminal end, an area of contusion and hemorrhagic necrosis measuring 2.5 × 2.0 cm covers most of the superior surface of the right cerebellar hemisphere and extends 5 mm over the midline. Beneath this area of contusion and communicating with the penetrating wound, a recent hematoma is found that measures 2.5 × 2.0 cm. The hemorrhage involves the region of the declivis, folium, and tuber. Smaller satellite contusions and hemorrhagic necrosis are scattered lateral to the large contusion of the superior surface of the cerebellum. Both cerebellar hemispheres are markedly swollen with flattened gyri and with a cerebellar pressure cone. Two small areas of hemorrhagic necrosis, each 3 mm in diameter, are present in the cortex of the herniated left cerebellar tonsil. The right cerebellar tonsil shows a single area of cortical hemorrhagic necrosis, also 3 mm in diameter.

An elliptical groove over the superior surface of the anterior lobe of the cerebellum indicates upward herniation of these structures through the incisura of the tentorium cerebelli. Horizontal sections of the cerebellum reveal the penetrating wound and the hemorrhage described above. These lesions have destroyed much of the cortex and subcortical white matter of the right cerebellar hemisphere, the dentate nuclei and probably the roof nuclei.

E. Brain stem
    The ventral surface of the pons and medulla is markedly flattened:
    The periaqueductal gray matter contains multiple petechial hemorrhages
    extending over an area of 8 to 9 mm in width on the left side and about 5
    mm on the right side. In sections above the pons, the midbrain reveals
    several irregular hemorrhages within the tegmentum. The largest of these
    hemorrhages is slitlike, measures 5 × 1 mm in size, and is situated in the
    left lateral tegmentum. Numerous petechial hemorrhages are found
    throughout both the tegmental and ventral portions of the rostral ¾ of the
    pons on multiple horizontal sections. Section through the medulla shows
    an area of hemorrhagic necrosis 4 × 3 mm in diameter located in the left
    inferior olive.
F. Ventricular system
    The lateral and third ventricles are moderately narrowed in size. They
    contain a small amount of blood clot totaling about 6 cc. The source of the
    intraventricular hemorrhage is due to rupture into the right inferior horn of
    the hemorrhage of the right temporal lobe. The fourth ventricle also con-
    tains a small amount of fresh blood clots.
G. Spinal cord and spinal canal
    The foramen magnum and the upper cervical vertebrae are inspected and
    they show no abnormalities.
    The bodies of the lower cervical, thoracic, and upper lumbar vertebrae
    are removed in a column. After inspecting the spinal nerve roots, the cervi-
    cal, thoracic, and lumbar spinal cord is removed in toto.
    A 41-cm portion of the spinal cord extending from the high cervical
    region into the lumbar region is examined. The leptomeninges are thin and
    transparent. The anterior spinal artery is thin-walled and shows no evi-
    dence of occlusion or laceration. The posterior aspect of the spinal cord
    additionally reveals thin leptomeninges and normal distribution of vessels
    and nerve roots. There is no evidence of pathologic damage to the spinal
    cord. The subarachnoid space shows faint blood staining. Multiple trans-
    verse sections of the spinal cord and nerve roots show no gross lesions.
H. Pituitary gland
    The diaphragma sella and pituitary stalk are normal in appearance. The
    pituitary gland measures 1.1 × 0.8 × 0.5 cm. Section shows a pink
    homogeneous anterior lobe and a reddish gray posterior lobe. The bony
    structures forming and surrounding the pituitary fossa are all within nor-
    mal limits.

MICROSCOPIC REPORT (NEUROPATHOLOGY)

There are 31 slides divided into three groups: A, B, and C. Each group is
again numbered as A-1, A-2, A-3, or B-1, B-2, B-3, B-4 and C-1, C-2, C-3, C-4,
etc.

Sections confirmed all the lesions described at the gross examination. All
tissue sections show congestion and some extravasation with occasional actual
petechial hemorrhages, the latter being particularly noticeable in the thalami
near the ventricular walls. A few mononuclear cells are present in the perivascular spaces. The ground substance of the cerebral cortex and centrum shows fine
vacuolations. In the occipital cortex, there is early status spongiosus, portions of
which have a laminar distribution. Some nerve cells have pyknotic nuclei and
homogenization of the cytoplasm, the latter showing definite eosinophilia. The

white matter of the frontal lobe shows occasional areas of pallid staining. In the ventral pons there is early necrosis in addition to the hemorrhages.

A-1, Right Frontal Lobe:
This section shows marked congestion of the meningeal and parenchymal blood vessels. The endothelium of the blood vessels shows hypertrophy. There is no inflammatory infiltrate in the meninges. There is a diffuse rarefaction of the matrix of the cortex and white matter, but more marked in the white matter where there are actual areas of early status spongiosus. Many of the nerve cells are pyknotic. The glial and ependymal elements are swollen.

A-2, Left Frontal Lobe:
Findings are similar to A-1 except that the status spongiosus of the white matter is not obvious.

A-3, Right Temporal Lobe—Hippocampus:
Findings are similar to A-2.

A-4, Left Temporal Lobe—Hippocampus:
In addition to similar findings as in A-3, there are several small petechiae in the cortex. This section also shows slight subarachnoid hemorrhage.

A-5, Right Parietal Lobe:
The general findings of these sections are similar to A-2. However, some nerve cells are not only pyknotic but are also beginning to show eosinophilia of the contracted and homogenized cytoplasm.

A-6, Left Parietal Lobe:
This slide shows findings similar to A-2. In addition, there is subarachnoid hemorrhage.

A-7, Right Occipital Lobe:
This section shows marked congestion of all the blood vessels with extravasation of blood in the white matter. The cortex shows early status spongiosus which has a suggestive laminar pattern.

A-8, Left Occipital Lobe:
This section shows findings similar to A-7 above. Some of the nerve cells are beginning to show eosinophilia of the cytoplasm.

A-9, Right Striatum:
In general the blood vessels and nerve cells show changes of the cortex similar to those described in A-2. The subependymal blood vessels show a few mononuclear cells in the perivascular spaces. There is also some extravasation of blood from these vessels.

A-10, Left Striatum:
These findings are similar to A-9.

A-11, Right Lenticular Nucleus:
The findings are similar to A-9 except the extravasation of blood is not obvious.

A-12, Left Lenticular Nucleus:
The findings are similar to A-11.

A-13, Right Thalamus:
These sections show generalized congestion and actual petechial hemorrhages in the walls of the third ventricle. The nerve cells show pyknotic changes. Portions of the matrix show early status spongiosus.

A-14, Left Thalamus:
The findings are similar to A-13, but the petechial hemorrhages are not as marked.

A-15, -16, -17, and -18, Spinal Cord:
Sections are taken from the cervical, thoracic, and lumbosacral regions. The vascular changes in the meninges and spinal cord are minimal and certainly not as pronounced as those in the cerebrum. A few of the nerve cells in the gray matter, mostly in anterior horns, show pyknotic changes.

B-1, Right Transverse Sinus:
Sections show red blood cells between the laminae of the dura. The sinus contains antemortem thrombus along the vessel walls. This thrombus consists mainly of platelets. In the remainder of the blood clot there are numerous neutrophils.

B-2, Right Sigmoid Sinus:
Portions of the dura show coagulation necrosis with tinctorial changes toward basophilia. Antemortem thrombus is also found in the sinus, as in B-1.

B-3, Right Frontal Lobe—Orbital Gyri:
Sections show hemorrhagic necrosis of the cortex.

B-4, Right Temporal Lobe—Parahippocampal and Fusiform Gyri:
This section shows most extensive hemorrhagic defects, both in the gray and white matter. The defect communicates with the external surface. The remaining portions of the specimen show changes similar to A-2.

B-5, Right Temporal Lobe:
The findings are similar to B-4.

B-6, Right Occipital Lobe, Medial Inferior Aspect:
Sections show superficial hemorrhagic defect of the cortex.

C-1, Left Inferior Temporal Lobe:
This section shows multiple hemorrhagic necrosis in the cortex.

C-2, Midbrain:
Section shows multiple hemorrhages. The cerebral aqueduct is patent.

C-3 and C-4, Pons:
Sections show multiple hemorrhage, mostly in the ventral portions, and acute necrosis. The fourth ventricle is collapsed.

C-5, Medulla:
Focal hemorrhagic necrosis is present in the left inferior olive.

C-6, Cerebellum, Dorsal Aspect:
This shows a large hemorrhagic defect with multiple petechial hemorrhages in portions of the dentate nucleus. In another portion of the dentate nucleus, where there is no hemorrhage, there is acute necrosis.

C-7, Cerebellum, Tonsil:
This shows multiple petechiae in the cortex.
Additional Microscopic Slides (Neuropathology): The pineal gland shows a few corpora amylacea.
Sections of the temporal lobe reveal essentially the same histopathologic findings described previously.
Slide Labeled Gunshot Wound (GSW #1), (Entrance Wound): The perpendicular section, stained with hematoxylin and eosin, through the wound track shows loss of epithelium and patchy areas of swollen dermis.
The area of margins of squamous epithelium shows perinuclear vacuolation and spindle form distortion.
The dermis is extensively involved with coagulation, also visible in special stain. The hair follicles and sebaceous glands are partly involved also.
Capillaries are dilated. There are areas of extravasation and infiltration by acute inflammatory cells. Scattered, varying-sized powder residues are found in the keratin layer and the inner surface of the wound track to a depth of 2 mm. There are also disclike powder granules embedded in the epidermis, and the powder-embedded area is surrounded by the pink-staining denatured collagen. Powder residues are in an assortment of shapes and sizes, the edges showing minute crystalloid material, which is also visible on the unstained sections.
Subcutaneous tissue and muscle elements are hemorrhagic and heavily infiltrated by neutrophils.
Microscopic diagnosis: Entry of the gunshot wound is consistent with very close range shooting.
Slide from Posterior Aspect of Helix of Right Ear, Including Grossly Described Powder Smudging and Tattooing: The sections stained with hematoxylin and eosin show patchy areas of loss of epithelium due to thermal and blast effect. The squamous epithelium between the exposed coagulated dermis shows perinuclear vacuolation and nuclear elongation, along with fragmentation at the edges.
Dark brown to black powder residues in varying sizes are embedded through the epithelium to the dermis, which is also recognizable in unstained sections. The dermis shows extensive coagulation of the collagen tissue. Sweat glands and hair follicles, together with associated sebaceous glands, are involved, with changes consistent with heat and blast effect. Coagulation of the collagen tissue is also visible on sections stained by Masson's method.

REPORTS OF X-RAY STUDIES

Description of Preoperative X-rays

Anteroposterior and lateral portable films of the skull, exposed on June 5, 1968, at approximately 1:00 A.M., reveal a gunshot wound of the right temporal bone. The wound of entry is 2.0 cm above the temporal tip and approximately midway between the external auditory canal and the sigmoid sinus region, approximately 1.0 cm posterior to the auditory canal.

There are two bullet tracks. One extends slightly anterior to the vertical dimension (15 degrees). The second extends 30 degrees posterior to the vertical dimension, so that the two tracks diverge 45 degrees.

In the frontal projection, both tracks extend superiorly toward the vertex at an angle of 30 degrees to the horizontal.

In the tracks of the bullet wound are numerous metallic foreign bodies and fragments of the mastoid. The largest metallic fragment is situated in the petrous ridge at about the arcuate eminence. This measures 12 mm in transverse dimension, 7 mm in vertical dimension, and approximately 12 mm in anteroposterior dimension.

Several metallic foreign bodies are present in the soft tissues lateral to the mastoid process. Twelve metallic foreign bodies, 1 mm or larger, are present in the mastoid process. In addition to the largest fragment described, at least thirty metallic fragments 1 mm or larger are present in the posterior fossa.

One fragment of bone and several metallic fragments projected through the orbit above the petrous ridge are, I believe, supratentorial, and in the mesial aspect of the temporal lobe posteriorly. A fragment, 7 mm in transverse diameter, 4 mm in greatest anteroposterior dimension and vertical dimension, is situated superiorly slightly to the left of the midline and 4.0 cm anterior to the inner cortex of the occipital bone at or just below the tentorium. The main fragments of the bullet are anterior to the sigmoid sinus as seen in the lateral projection, and this includes the major bony fragment as well.

Description of Postmortem Radiographs

Postmortem radiographs exposed at 2:00 A.M. to 3:00 A.M., under the direction of the Chief Medical Examiner-Coroner, on June 6, 1968, reveal that a major portion of the petrous ridge has been removed, together with most of the metallic foreign bodies and the detached osseous fragments.

At this time, the metallic fragment most superior and posterior has shifted slightly posteriorly and to the right.

Small fragments remain in the soft tissues lateral to the temporal bone, numbering approximately eleven and very minute. Other fragments, approximately seven in number, are situated directly above the petrous apex and, I believe, supratentorial, in the temporal lobe. This represents the remains of the largest metallic fragment noted preoperatively. Other minute fragments are present in the posterior fossa, numbering approximately twenty.

All of the bony fragments have been removed.

X-rays of the skull at the conclusion of the postmortem revealed that five minute metallic foreign bodies were present in the skin, and approximately twenty minute fragments remained embedded in the remaining portion of the temporal bone in the region of the semicircular canals.

Description of Specimen Radiograph of Surgical Bony Specimen

A series of x-ray films was obtained on June 7, 1968, between 4:00 P.M. and 7:30 P.M.

The initial x-rays consisted of the fragments of temporal bone removed at surgery. These were exposed on industrial film-type M (Kodak) and reveal many more minute metallic foreign bodies than were evident on the early films. Pieces of bone identifiable as mastoid process are filled with approximately 70 individual metallic fragments. Others bearing the Rongeur marks are fragments of cortex removed at surgery from the craniotomy site. Other fragments represent petrous ridge and are also embedded with innumerable fine metallic particles.

The specimen of temporal bone removed at postmortem includes the craniotomy site and the remaining portion of the mastoid process extending posteriorly to include the lateral sinus groove and the facial canal distally. Mesially, the bone is amputated lateral to the cochlea. This contains the external auditory canal. Posterior and superior to the canal are many metallic fragments. These number at least sixty, the majority less than 1 mm in size, with ten above 1 mm.

Description of Specimen X-rays Exposed at the Good Samaritan Hospital (Friday, June 7, 1968)

X-rays of the entire brain, taken initially in the vertex-base direction, reveal small metallic foreign bodies in the cerebellum and temporal lobe. There is a considerable defect of the cerebellum on the right. A small amount of residual contrast (Hypaque) is present in the arterial tree in the left temporal area.

Following the above, the individual sections were x-rayed and labeled respectively: A for the tips of the frontal lobes and successively posteriorly at 2.0 cm intervals, B; C (which includes the anterior aspect of the temporal lobes); and D; etc. E shows one metallic foreign body in the right temporal lobe, plus a defect in the mesial aspect of the temporal lobe in the region of the uncal gyrus. Residual contrast is in the choroid plexus of the lateral ventricle on the left.

Specimen labeled F consists of slice F plus the separate specimen F-1 from the temporal lobe, which contains ten minute metallic foreign bodies in one segment and three minute ones in another area. The cerebellum is also present which reveals a large defect and twenty minute metallic foreign bodies. The specimens of the brain, G and H, extending to the occipital pole, reveal no abnormality. Separate x-rays were performed on specimen F and F-1 and the cerebellum, plus x-rays of the meninges. The meninges are tattooed with many metallic foreign bodies surrounding the defect, which is in the region of the original wound of entry.

These number fully fifty, with all but three or four under 1 mm in diameter.

Description of Skin and Hair X-rays

X-rays of 68-5731 obtained at the Good Samaritan Hospital between 1:00 and 3:00 P.M, Saturday, June 8, 1968.

The right ear is portrayed in profile and en face. The profile shows the skin surface directed away from the identifying number. The larger side of the ear specimen is to the right in both projections.

Tattooed in the skin are many small metallic foreign bodies. Other foreign bodies are present in the ear which do not appear to be metallic.

Gunshot Wound No. 1 was examined in profile with the cutaneous surface directed toward the number. Two fragments of the wound are present. Both reveal metallic foreign bodies of varying size from barely visible to 1 mm in diameter in the subcutaneous tissue. Many minute foreign bodies are present in the skin superficially surrounding the wound of entry. These resemble in size the particles seen in the ear.

The skin of Gunshot Wound No. 2 and Gunshot Wound No. 3 also reveals the superficial dense metallic impregnation of the skin with several metallic foreign bodies in the subcutaneous tissue. These specimens are also arranged in profile with the cutaneous surface extending toward the identifying number.

The third examination is of the scalp hair obtained prior to surgery. In this area, many dustlike metallic particles are evident, varying in size but all extremely small and differing appreciably from the several artifacts noticed to the left of the label "scalp hair" on the superior aspect of the film.

Three metallic particles are noted in the hair obtained at autopsy. Two of these are extremely minute and one is approximately 0.5 mm in diameter.

Description of X-Rays of Skin Wounds

X-rays were obtained of the skin wounds, which are labeled 1, 2, and 3.

Gunshot Wound No. 1:
A profile view of the skin surrounding wound of entry in the right mastoid area reveals a few metallic foreign bodies superficially and other larger foreign bodies (1 cm) in the subcutaneous tissue.

Gunshot Wounds Nos. 2 and 3:
A frontal projection of the axillary skin surrounding wounds labeled 2 and 3 reveals fine metallic foreign bodies in both these situations. The wound of exit is placed in profile. Wound 2 reveals two minute metallic foreign bodies barely visible in the subcutaneous tissue below the wound.

HEAD AND NERVOUS SYSTEM (GENERALLY)

Also revealed by the reflection of the scalp is a fairly well demarcated area of nonrecent hemorrhagic discoloration, about 1.5 cm in greatest dimension, in the left parietal occipital region. No associated galeal hemorrhage is demonstrated.

The cerebrospinal fluid is blood tinged.

Abundant and freshly clotted, but drying blood is found at the right external auditory canal, extending outward to the lateral interstices of the external ear. No evidence of hemorrhage is found at the left ear.

The spinal cord is taken for further evaluation. At the time of removal of the cord, a small amount of cervical epidural hemorrhage is noted. There is no evidence on preliminary inspection of avulsion of roots leading to the right brachial plexus.

Those portions of peripheral nervous system exposed by the described dissection show no abnormality.

Gunshot Wound No. 2
GROSS
This is a through-and-through wound of the right axillary, medial shoulder, and anterior superior chest areas, excluding the thorax proper. The wound of entry is centered 12½ inches (31.8 cm) from the vertex, 9 inches (22.9 cm) to the right of midline, and 3¾ inches (8.3 cm) from the back (anterior to a coronal plane passing through the surface of the skin at the scapula region). There is a regularly elliptical defect ³/₁₆ × ⅛ inch overall (about 0.5 × 0.3 cm) with thin rim of abrasion. There is no apparent charring or powder residue in the adjacent and subjacent tissue. The subcutaneous fatty tissue is hemorrhagic.

The wound path is through soft tissue, medially to the left, superiorly and somewhat anteriorly. Bony structures, major blood vessels, and the brachial plexus have been spared.

The exit wound is centered 9¾ inches (about 24.5 cm) from the vertex and about 5 inches (about 12.5 cm) to the right of midline anteriorly in the infra-clavicular region. There is a nearly circular defect slightly less than ¼ × ³/₁₆ inch overall (0.6 × 0.5 cm). Orientation of the wounds of entry and exit is such that their major axes at the skin surfaces coincide with the central axis of a probe passed along the entirety of the wound path. No evidence of deflection of trajectory is found.

MICROSCOPIC EXAMINATION OF THE SLIDE LABELED GUNSHOT WOUND NO. 2 (GSW #2) ENTRANCE WOUND

The perpendicular sections of the gunshot wound show cellular degeneration of the margins of the covering epithelium. The dermis shows extensive coagulation, early cell infiltration by mostly neutrophiles, and hemolyzed and relatively intact erythrocytes. The area of coagulation necrosis includes disintegration of apparently sweat and sebaceous gland. Only remnants are visualized. Gunpowder granules embedded into the dermis and the surface of the gunshot wound track are visible on stained and unstained sections. The subcutaneous and adipose tissue shows extensively extravasated hemorrhage.

Gunshot Wound No. 3
GROSS

The wound of entry is centered 14 inches (35.6 cm) from the vertex and 8½ inches (21.6 cm) to the right of midline, 2 inches (5 cm) from the back anterior to a plane pasing through the skin surface overlying the scapula, and ½ inch (1.2 cm) posterior to the mid-axillary line. There is a nearly circular defect ³/₁₆ inch by slightly more than ⅛ inch overall (0.5 × 0.4 cm). There is a thin marginal abrasion rim without evidence of charring or apparent residue in the adjacent skin or subjacent soft tissue. The subcutaneous fatty tissue is hemorrhagic.

The wound path is directed medially to the left, superiorly and posteriorly through soft tissue of the medial portion of the axilla and soft tissue of the upper back, terminating at a point at the level of the 6th thoracic vertebra as close as about ½ inch (1.2 cm) to the right of midline.

BULLET RECOVERY

A deformed bullet (later identified as .22 caliber) is recovered at the terminus of the wound path just described at 8:40 A.M., June 6, 1968. There is a unilateral, transverse deformation, the contour of which is indicated on an accompanying diagram. The initials, TN, and the numbers 31 are placed on the base of the bullet for future identification. The usual evidence envelope is prepared. The bullet, so marked and so enclosed as evidence, is given to Sergeant W. Jordan, No. 7167, Rampart Detectives, Los Angeles Police Department, at 8:49 A.M. this date for further studies.

An irregularly bordered and somewhat elliptical zone of variably mottled recent ecchymosis is present in the superior-medial axillary skin on the right, in the zones of wounds of entry No. 2 and No. 3, especially the former. The ecchymosis measures 3½ × 1½ inches (9 × 3.8 cm) overall with the right upper extremity extended completely upward (longitudinally).

Triangulation of Gunshot Wounds

Angles and planes refer to the body considered in the standing position, in accordance with usual anatomic custom.

GUNSHOT WOUND NO. 1

Goniometric studies by Dr. Scanlan are described by him elsewhere in this report. Photographs of internal features of the skull are confirmatory.

GUNSHOT WOUND NO. 2

Autopsy measurements indicate an angle of 35 degrees counterclockwise from the transverse plane as viewed frontally. Triangulation measurements from photographs give an angle of 33 degrees.

Autopsy measurements indicate an angle of 59 degrees counterclockwise from the transverse plane as viewed laterally from the right. Measurements from photographs also indicate an angle of 59 degrees.

Autopsy measurements indicate an angle of 25 degrees measured clockwise from the coronal plane (anteriorly) as viewed from the vertex.

GUNSHOT WOUND NO. 3

Autopsy measurements show an angle of 30 degrees upward from the transverse plane, counterclockwise as viewed frontally. Photographic studies also show an angle of 30 degrees.

Autopsy measurements show an angle of 67 degrees clockwise from the transverse plane as viewed laterally from the right. Photographs indicate an angle of about 70 degrees.

Measurements indicate an angle of 5½ degrees counterclockwise and behind the coronal plane as viewed from the vertex. The photographs are in agreement for this small angle.

FINAL SUMMARY

Gunshot Wound No. 1 (Fatal Gunshot Wound)

ENTRY:	Right mastoid region
COURSE:	Skin of right mastoid region, right mastoid, petrous portion of right temporal bone, right temporal lobe, and right hemisphere of cerebellum
EXIT:	None
DIRECTION:	Right to left, slightly to front, upward
BULLET RECOVERY:	Fragments (see text)

LESIONS IN DETAIL (NEUROPATHOLOGY)

A. Primary lesions—caused by the bullet and further injuries by bone and bullet fragments
1. Bone, dura, and dural sinus
    a. Penetration of right mastoid process
    b. Fracture of right petrous ridge
    c. Severance of right petrosal sinus
    d. Metal fragments in right temporal bone
2. Cerebrum
    a. Contusion-laceration and hemorrhage of right temporal lobe
    b. Intraventricular hemorrhage due to above
    c. Metal and bone fragments in right temporal lobe
3. Cerebellum
    a. Hemorrhagic tract and cavity in right cerebellar hemisphere
    b. Metal and bone fragments in right cerebellar hemisphere

B. Immediate Secondary lesions
   1. Bone Lesion
      a. Fracture of right supraorbital plate
   2. Meningeal Lesions
      a. Subdural hemorrhage
      b. Subarachnoid hemorrhage
      c. Laceration of right supraorbital dura
   3. Cerebral Lesions
      a. Contusion-laceration of right orbital gyri
      b. Contusion-laceration of right occipital lobe
      c. Contusion of contralateral (left) inferior temporal gyrus
   4. Cerebellum
      a. Hemorrhagic necrosis of cerebellar tonsils
   5. Brain Stem
      a. Hemorrhage in midbrain
      b. Hemorrhagic necrosis of left inferior olive of medulla
   6. Epidural hemorrhage of C1 and C2 vertebral level
C. Later Secondary Lesions
   1. Edema of brain and herniations
   2. Subdural hemorrhage
   3. Subarachnoid hemorrhage
   4. Intracerebral and intraventricular hemorrhage
   5. Hemorrhagic infarction of right temporal cortex
   6. Intracerebellar and intraventricular hemorrhage
   7. Petechial hemorrhages of thalami
   8. Brain stem hemorrhage and early necrosis
   9. Herniation of cerebellum through craniotomy wound
   10. Early laminar necrosis of occipital lobe

Gunshot Wound No. 2, Through-and-Through

ENTRY:	Right axillary region
COURSE:	Soft tissue of right axilla and right infraclavicular region
EXIT:	Right infraclavicular region
DIRECTION:	Right to left, back to front, upward
BULLET RECOVERY:	None

Gunshot Wound No. 3

ENTRY:	Right axillary region (just below Gunshot Wound No. 2 entry)
COURSE:	Soft tissue of right axilla, soft tissue of right upper back to the level of the 6th cervical vertebra just beneath the skin
EXIT:	None
DIRECTION:	Right to left, back to front, upward
BULLET RECOVERY:	.22 caliber bullet from the soft tissue of paracervical region at level of 6th cervical vertebra at 8:40 A.M., June 6, 1968

Evidence of Recent Surgical Procedures
   1. Craniotomy, right temporal occipital
   2. Other, minor surgical procedures are described elsewhere
Pathologic Findings Related to Gunshot Wound No. 1

1. Hypostatic Pneumonia
Miscellaneous Pathologic Findings not Related to cause of Death
  1. Adenoma of the left kidney (benign)
  2. Retention cyst of left kidney

Portions of the text on John and Robert Kennedy in this chapter are repro-
duced from Noguchi, in Wecht, Legal Medicine Annual 1973. Courtesy of
Appleton-Century-Crofts, Publishing Division of Prentice-Hall, Inc., En-
glewood Cliffs, N.J. Portions of the text on Abraham Lincoln are reproduced
from Lattimer, J. K.: The wound that killed Lincoln. Illinois Medical Journal,
138:514, 1970.

REFERENCES

1. Brooks, S. M.: Our Murdered Presidents—The Medical Story, New York, Frederick Fell, 1966.
2. Knight, J. M. (ed.): 3 Assassinations—The Deaths of John and Robert Kennedy and Martin Luther King. New York, Facts on File, 1971.
3. Lattimer, G., Lattimer, J. K. and Lattimer, J.: The Kennedy-Connally one bullet theory. Resident and Staff Physician, 20:33, 1974.
4. Lattimer, J. K.: Observations based on a review of the autopsy photographs, x-rays, and related materials of the late President John F. Kennedy. Medical Times, 100:34, 1972.
5. ———.: The wound that killed Lincoln. Illinois Medical Journal, 138:514, 1970. Original autopsy report in Surgeon General's Office, Washington, D.C. April 15, 1885.
6. Noguchi, T. Postmortem protocols in official medical-legal investigation—a study in contrast (Autopsy reports in the assassination deaths of President John F. Kennedy and Senator Robert F. Kennedy). In Wecht, C. H. (ed.): Legal Medicine Annual 1973. New York, Appleton-Century-Crofts, 1973.
7. Report of the President's Commission on the Assassination of President Kennedy. U.S. Government Printing Office, Washington, D.C., 1964.
8. Wecht, C. H. and Smith, R. P.: Medical Evidence in the Assassination of President John F. Kennedy. In Wecht, C. H. (ed.): Legal Medicine Annual 1974. New York, Appleton-Century-Crofts, 1974.

17

Current Research in the Investigation of Shooting Cases

Research in the areas related to the investigation of crimes committed with firearms has been sporadic in the current century. The use of the comparison microscope contributed greatly to the science of forensic ballistics. During the years around the second World War considerable amount of work was done to determine the chemical composition of firearms discharge residue, powders, primers, lubricants, bullets and fouling.[7,23] In recent years, researchers have concentrated more on the problem of detection of gunshot residues on human skin and on clothing. Neutron activation analysis and atomic absorption spectrometry have gained popularity as research tools to study gunshot residues. Scanning electron microscopy has been applied to study bullets and cartridge cases. These and other modern methods are reviewed in this chapter. In order to put the current research efforts in proper perspective, some of the previous work is briefly cited first.

EARLIER WORK ON GUNSHOT RESIDUE

For detection of gunshot residue on clothing Walker[23] has described a test which can be performed as follows:

Desensitize a glossy photographic paper by fixing it in hypo bath for 15 to 20 minutes. Then wash it thoroughly for about 45 minutes, and dry it. Immerse the dried paper in a warm 5 percent solution of sulfanilic acid and leave there for 10 minutes. Allow it to dry. Then dip the paper in 0.5 percent solution of alpha-naphthylamine in methyl alcohol and dry again. Place the paper so prepared on a pad of cloth on top of a flat surface. The fabric to be examined for powder pattern should then be laid flat with the side suspected to have gunpowder in contact with the paper. Next, place a layer of cloth moistened with 20 percent acetic acid over the fabric to be examined and press the whole pack with a warm electric iron for 5-10 minutes. Remove the paper and wash it with hot water and methyl alcohol. If nitrite is present it will be seen as bright orange-red spots on the paper.

247

This test is specific for nitrites produced by the combustion of gunpowder. It is reliable and hence it is widely used. Examination of the evidence clothing and of similar clothing showing patterns of test fires made with evidence weapon and ammunition will allow comparison of powder patterns. A permanent graphic documentation is possible by this test without altering or destroying the evidence clothing. Further, photographs of the test results can be made for convenient filing and later use in court. An additional advantage of this test is that the blood stains do not cause interference.

The paraffin test (described in Chapter 10), which relies on color change to detect the presence of nitrite and nitrate, was being used to detect gunshot residue. This test is unreliable and has fallen into disrepute because it is non-specific.

In 1959, Harrison and Gilroy described simple tests for the detection of antimony, barium and lead in gunshot residue on human skin.[6] The procedure consists of the following steps:

1. Removal of the residue with a piece of white cotton cloth moistened with 0.1 molar hydrochloric acid
2. Addition of 1 or 2 drops of 10-per-cent alcoholic solution of triphenylarsonium on the piece of cloth (An orange ring on the cloth developing in two minutes indicates positive test for antimony.)
3. Addition of 2 drops of freshly prepared 5-per-cent solution of sodium rhodizonate to the center of the orange ring (Development of red color inside of orange ring is positive test for barium, or lead, or both barium and lead.)
4. Addition of 1 or 2 drops of hydrochloric acid to red-colored area on the cloth dried after step 3 (Development of blue color inside the orange ring is confirmation of test for lead, and persistence of red color in the center of the orange ring is confirmation of test for antimony.)

This test is an improvement over the paraffin test because it is specific for antimony, barium and lead.

NEUTRON ACTIVATION ANALYSIS AND ATOMIC ABSORPTION SPECTROMETRY

Neutron activation analysis and atomic absorption spectrometry have proven to be of help in the investigation of shooting cases. The work done in recent years indicates that they can aid in (1) identifying holes in clothing, tissue, wood, etc. as bullet holes from the presence of lead, antimony, barium and copper; (2) determining the range of fire from concentration pattern of antimony around the bullet hole; (3) determining common origin of bullet fragments or shotgun pellets found at different places from the concentrations of lead, antimony, arsenic, copper and silver in these alloys; and (4) determining from the presence of lead, antimony and barium on hands whether or not a person has fired a gun. Analytical procedures developed for these applications, have been detailed by Krishnan.[16]

Neutron Activation Analysis (NAA)

NAA is a chemical method for analysis of elements in many materials. It is based on the detection and measurement of characteristic radioisotopes formed by irradiation in a nuclear reactor. The atoms of the elements present in a specimen are bombarded with neutrons. Some of the nuclei of the atoms capture neutrons. Those atoms capturing neutrons become radioactive. The radioactivity is measured with a detector connected to an analyzer.

The method is being extensively used in biological, physical, environmental and forensic sciences. Here we are only concerned with the review of its uses in the investigation of shooting cases.

The advantages of NAA technique are that it is effective in determining the firing distances much beyond the range of other procedures and it is one of the most effective techniques for the detection of antimony and barium in gunshot residues. The NAA technique is not without drawbacks, however. It is expensive, time consuming and not readily available. Also, it is not effective in detecting lead, which is one of the important constituents of gunshot residue.[12] Another factor discouraging greater use of NAA is the troublesome work of postirradiation radiochemical separations. There is hope, however, for minimizing this problem. Rudzitis and Wahlgren have developed a technique that eliminates postirradiation radiochemistry.[21] Also, by this technique the sample size is reduced to enable irradiation of over 100 samples at one time.

Determination of Range of Fire by NAA. The need for a technique of accurate determination of the firing distance in crimes with firearms, especially when powder residues are not detectable by conventional methods, has stimulated some researchers to seek advances in this area. The technique of NAA was used by Krishnan for this purpose in 1967.[13] He demonstrated that the concentration patterns of the metallic residue deposited around bullet holes can be used to determine the distance of fire. Krishnan reported further data on the concentration patterns of antimony ("the constituent of the bullet which is most easily detected by NAA") deposited around bullet holes and indicated that NAA can help determine shooting distances with a deviation of $\pm$ 2 inches.[15] The method used by Krishnan consisted of the following steps:

1. Test firing using the same target, ammunition and weapon, as in the case under investigation.
2. Removal of circular portions of target areas.
3. Activation of these portions in a nuclear reactor.
4. Quantitative estimation of antimony by gamma ray scintillation spectrometry after waiting for a few days.
5. Determination of distances of fire by comparison of test shots.

Examination of Gunshot Residues on Hands by NAA.   The detection of lead and antimony on a hand could indicate that the hand has fired a gun. The differences in the concentrations of lead and antimony are such that they form a good basis for the conclusion as to whether one of the hands has fired a gun.[17] The samples can be simply taken by washing the hands with 5 to 10 per cent nitric acid and examined for antimony by NAA. As an alternative, the cellulose "film-lift" method described by Pillay and his associates may be used for the collection of gunshot residues.[19] Krishnan and associates indicate that on unwashed hands such as in suicides the deposits are present for at least 48 hours and mild washing of the hand does not remove the deposits completely. Krishnan has observed more recently that with normal activity the gunshot residues remain on the hand for up to 17 hours.[12] Kilty's observations are different, however.[11] He noted that there was loss or decrease of antimony and barium from the hands following physical activity by the shooter. His experiments involving various activities by the shooter such as washing of hands, rinsing of hands, wiping of hands with towel, placing of hands in pockets and unrestricted activity except washing of hands lead him to believe that no meaningful information can be obtained from NAA of swabs obtained from hands of a suspected shooter if he engages in some degree of activity.

Atomic Absorption Spectrometry (AAS)

Atomic absorption spectrometry is a quantitative analytical technique for the determination of small concentrations of metals in a variety of materials. The sample to be examined is usually in solution or suspension. By this technique the analyst can measure the absorption of a specific wavelength of light by the sample to be examined. The degree of absorption is related to the concentration of the element in solution by use of calibrating standards. Since the wavelength bands that are absorbed by each element are narrow and specific for different elements, identification and quantitation of various elements is possible. The machine used is called an atomic absorption spectrophotometer.

The working of an atomic absorption spectrophotometer is simple. The sample to be examined is heated to a high temperature by burning in a flame. The flame causes breakdown of the chemical bonds between the molecules. This breakup of chemical bonds enables individual atoms to float freely in the area of the sample. Individual atoms can absorb ultraviolet or visible radiation of specific wavelengths. The source of light is generally a hollow cathode lamp that emits a spectrum of the element of interest. A monochromator isolates a resonance line of the lamp's spectrum and the intensity of this line is measured by a photodetector. When the light is passed through the flame, a certain portion of the light is absorbed by the atoms of the element looked for. A comparison of decrease in the intensity of the resonance line resulting from the absorption of the sample can be made with absorption produced by a standard of known concentration. The comparison will give the concentration of the element of interest.

The application of atomic absorption to chemical analysis began in 1955. Now, atomic absorption technique has wide applicability; it can determine the concentration of some 70 elements. It is highly sensitive, with precision in the range of 0.2 to 0.5 per cent. Sample preparation is easy, standardization is simple, and very little instruction is required to operate the instruments. Atomic absorption has few chemical and practically no spectral or excitation interferences and hence time-consuming chemical separations are usually unnecessary. Because of its sensitivity, low cost and easy availability, atomic absorption has attracted the attention of the criminologist and its use in the investigation of shooting cases is increasing.

Determination of Range of Fire by AAS.   AAS can be used to estimate the distance of fire by determining the concentration pattern of lead around bullet holes. A practical method based on experimental work has been outlined by Krishnan.[14] He conducted test fires using different weapons and various ammunitions on different target materials such as cloth, filter paper and human skin. He then examined circular target samples around the bullet holes with Perkin Elmer Model 303 unit atomic absorption spectrophotometer. The following conclusions were drawn from the experiments:

1. Accurate determinations of the distance of fire are possible on the basis of lead concentration pattern around bullet holes, the accuracy being ± 10 per cent.
2. Lead can be detected by AAS at firing distances of 36 inches. (By conventional methods powder residue around bullet holes is not detectable beyond 18 to 20 inches.)
3. The lead concentrations on filter paper target and human skin are similar, but they are slightly higher on cloth.
4. Different weapons produce somewhat different lead concentration patterns, but the general concentration range with different weapons fired from a fixed distance is similar.
5. Different ammunitions produce somewhat different lead concen-

tration patterns, but the error introduced by the use of different ammunitions in the determination of distance of fire is not significant.

Examination of Gunshot Residues on Hands by AAS. The difference in the concentration of lead as measured by AAS will help the investigator draw a conclusion as to whether a hand has fired a gun.[17] The samples of gunshot residues from hands can be obtained with cotton swabs dipped in 5 to 10 per cent nitric acid. By AAS and NAA it is possible to detect accurately small amounts of various elements such as antimony, arsenic, barium, copper and silver. These methods have increased the sensitivity and specificity of detection of various elements, especially antimony and barium, in shooting cases.

The excitation technique most commonly used is by flame vaporization. However, Stone and Petty have reported that the flame atomic absorption technique lacks sensitivity for barium and antimony and they suggest co-ordinated studies including soft x-ray radiography and non-flame AAS.[22] Renshaw and his colleagues have used non-flame AAS for quantitative estimation of lead, antimony and barium with good results.[20]

Other techniques recently used to analyze gunshot residues are reviewed below.

ELECTRODELESS PLASMA EMISSION SPECTROMETRY

This method has been used in the detection of gunshot residue only recently.[3] The method is capable of determining metals and metalloids at the ultratrace level in microlitre and microgram samples. It is also possible to make multielement determinations with minimal interelement effects. The technique is highly sensitive and has some advantages over the flame atomic absorption (Fassel and Kniseley, 1974).

CHARGED PARTICLE INDUCED X-RAY ANALYSIS

Barnes and his colleagues have suggested the use of charged particle induced x-ray analysis for the detection of various elements in gunshot residue.[1] This method also is sensitive for the detection of all elements in gunshot residue. However, the instrument is expensive and not easily available in crime laboratories.

PHOTOLUMINESCENCE TECHNIQUE

The molecular photoluminescence technique has been studied to detect metallic elements in gunshot residue.[8] In this method the hands of the person suspected to have fired the shot are washed in a stream of distilled water. The washing is then filtered and the residue collected on a membrane filter. When the residue is dissolved in hydrochloric acid, lead and antimony form chloride ion complexes that luminesce upon selective ultraviolet excitation at low temperature. The complexes emit light with maxima at wavelengths characteristic of the elements lead and antimony.

According to the investigators, this quantitative method is convenient and sensitive. It is capable of detecting as little as 1.0 ng of lead and 10 ng of antimony. The method is rapid: the total time for collection of the sample and its analysis is less than 30 minutes. It may be possible to use it as a screening test or presumptive test for the presence of gunshot residue on the hands. Further work with different guns and ammunition and analyses for barium and copper in gunshot residue using photoluminescence methods are planned by Jones and Nesbitt.

Gunshot residues present variable patterns. No matter what method of analysis is used, these patterns should be carefully interpreted. Many factors influence the pattern on the target. These factors, in order of importance, are distance of fire, length of barrel of gun, rate of burning of propellant, type of propellant, caliber of weapon, muzzle-target angle, target material, type of primer, weight of propellant and type of weapon.[2]

SCANNING ELECTRON MICROSCOPE ANALYSIS

Scanning electron microscopy (SEM) has been applied in recent years by forensic scientists to study, among other things, firearm markings.[18] This instrumental system is superior to optical microscopy because the depth of field and high resolution yield better details and because the entire field of study is in focus at one time. The work dealing with the study of firing pin impressions and microstriations on bullets is briefly reviewed here.

Comparison of Firing Pin Impressions

Pistols. In 1972, Grove and his colleagues reported that the scanning electron microscope was a significant tool for comparing firing pin impressions.[5] They examined firing impressions from 16 semiautomatic pistols. Fifty rounds were fired from each pistol. The first, second, tenth and in some cases the fiftieth firing pin impressions were examined in a scanning electron microscope (Model 700, Materials Analysis Co.) at a magnification of 50. For comparison, several firing pin impressions were also examined optically. The criterion considered necessary for a positive comparison between firing pin impressions was the presence of individualizing persistent details (four or more individual characteristics in addition to similar class characteristics) on all rounds fired. The examinations not only showed that the SEM was superior to optical microscopy but also indicated that it was consistent, because it identified the first and the fiftieth firing pin impressions from each series of several weapons.

Rifles and Shotguns.   After the successful application of SEM to the study of firing pin impressions from pistols, Grove and his colleagues extended their work to the study of firing pin impressions of shotguns and rifles.[4] They examined impressions from 12 autoejecting shotguns and rifles the same way they examined the firing pin impressions of the semiautomatic pistols. The criteria for making a positive comparison consisted, as with pistols, of four or more characteristics in addition to similar class characteristics. The first, second, tenth and in some instances the fiftieth firing pin impressions on cartridge cases were examined. These examinations revealed that 50 per cent of the shotgun impressions and 75 per cent of the rifle impressions could be matched on the basis of four or more individual characteristics. The ones that could not be matched were devoid of any impressions. The study further indicated that the impressions from one gun had no individual identifying features in common with those from any other weapon. The presence of pre-existing primer marks did not cause any artefacts and thus did not affect the comparison of firing pin impressions. The authors conclude that the scanning electron microscope is a useful instrument in identifying cartridge cases fired from rifles and shotguns.

Comparison of Bullets

A fired bullet has striations and microstriations along the shoulder of the land impressions. SEM has been applied to study these striations at magnifications higher than are achievable through an optical examination of the bullets. Judd and his associates examined the markings on two sets of copper-jacketed bullets by SEM.[9] They took photomicrographs of the striations to determine whether or not there was a consistent pattern of microstriations. Then they made a topographical comparative study of the microstriations with the aid of a comparative imaging system.[10] Photomicrographs were then made to record the images of each set of the microstriations in proper orientation. The examinations revealed that each striation on the shoulder of a land impression along a bullet had microstriations within it. These microstriations did not have a counterpart set on the same bullet. The striations on the land impression, excluding the shoulders, showed markings that were present only between one set of striations on one particular bullet. The authors indicate that the SEM examination can show a consistent set of microstriations within each striation in a manner that is not optically possible. It can thus allow direct comparison of bullets to the extent that "a determination of possible common origin could be made."

REFERENCES

1. Barnes, B. K., Beghian, L. E., Kegel, G. H. R., Mathur, S. C. and Quinn, P.: Charged particle induced x-ray analysis—A new tool in forensic science. J. Radioanalytical Chemistry, *15*:13, 1973.
2. Barnes, F. C. and Helson, R. A.: An empirical study of gunpowder residue patterns. J. For. Sci., *19*:448, 1974.
3. Fassel, V. A. and Kniseley, R. N.: Inductively coupled plasma-optical emission spectroscopy. Analytical Chemistry, *46*:1110A, 1974.
4. Grove, C. A., Judd, G. and Horn, R.: Evaluation of SEM potential in the examination of shotgun and rifle firing pin impressions. J. For. Sci., *19*:441, 1974.
5. ———: Examination of firing pin impressions by scanning electron microscopy. J. For. Sci., *17*:645, 1972.
6. Harrison, H. C. and Gilroy, R.: Firearms discharge residue. J. For. Sci., *4*:184, 1959.
7. Hatcher, J. S.: Textbook of Firearms Investigation, Identification and Evidence. Marines, Small-Arms Technical Publishing, 1935.
8. Jones, P. F. and Nesbitt, R. S.: A photoluminescence technique for detection of gunshot residue. J. For. Sci., *20*:231, 1975.
9. Judd, G., Sabo, J., Hamilton, W., Ferriss, S. and Horn, R.: SEM microstriation characterization of bullets and contaminant particle identification. J. For. Sci., *19*:798, 1974.
10. Judd, G., Wilson, R. and Weiss, H.: A topographical comparison imaging system for SEM applications. Sixth IITRI Symposium, p. 167. Chicago, IIT Research Institute, 1973.
11. Kilty, J. S.: Activity after shooting and its effect on the retention of primer residue. J. For. Sci., *20*:219, 1975.
12. Krishnan, S. S.: Detection of gunshot residue on the hands by neutron activation analysis and atomic absorption analysis. J. For. Sci., *19*:789, 1974.
13. ———: Determination of gunshot firing distances and identification of bullet holes by neutron activation analysis. J. For. Sci., *12*:112, 1967.
14. ———: Firing distance determination by atomic absorption spectrophotometry. J. For. Sci., *19*:351, 1974.
15. ———: Firing distance determination by neutron activation analysis. J. For. Sci., *12*:471, 1967.
16. ———: Trace element analysis by atomic absorption spectrometry and neutron activation analysis in the investigation of shooting cases. Canadian society of Forensic Science Journal, *6*:56, 1973.
17. Krishnan, S. S., Gillespie, K. A. and Anderson, E. J.: Rapid detection of firearm discharge residues by atomic absorption and neutron activation analysis. J. For. Sci., *16*:144, 1971.
18. MacDonell, H. L. and Pruden, L. H.: Application of scanning electron microscope to the examination of firearm markings. Scanning Electron Microscopy, 1971 Proceedings, p. 569. Chicago, IIT Research Institute, 1971.

19. Pillay, K. K. S., Jester, W. A., Fox, H. A.: New method for the collection and analysis of gunshot residues as forensic evidence. J. For. Sci., *19*:768, 1974.
20. Renshaw, G. D., Pounds, C. A. and Pearson, E. F.: Quantitative estimation of lead, antimony and barium in gunshot residues by the non-flame atomic absorption spectrophotometry. Atomic Absorption Newsletter, *12*:55, 1973.
21. Rudzitis, E. and Wahlgren, M.: Firearm residue detection by instrumental neutron activation analysis. J. For. Sci., *20*:119, 1975.
22. Stone, I. C. and Petty, C. S.: Examination of gunshot residues. J. For. Sci., *19*:784, 1974.
23. Walker, J. T.: Bullet holes and chemical residues in shooting cases. J. Crim. Law and Crim., *31*:497, 1940.

18

Preparation of Reports and Presentation of Evidence in Court

The importance of preparing meticulous, detailed and accurate reports of medicolegal investigation cannot be overemphasized. Lapses or inaccuracies in the reports and errors in presenting the evidence in court can undermine the investigative efforts and result in a serious miscarriage of justice. Therefore, every investigator preparing a medicolegal report must be careful in documenting the factual data and in formulating the opinions.

In cases of crimes committed with guns, the investigators most frequently involved are the police officer (detective), the pathologist and the firearms examiner. The reports prepared by these investigators and the presentation of evidence by them in court are discussed in this chapter.

PREPARATION OF REPORTS

The Police Investigator's Report

Preparation of a report of a criminal investigation is not always an easy task. The circumstances in each case are different and the degree of effort needed varies. The degree of involvement of one investigator in the various phases of investigation can also vary. For instance, a single individual may be responsible for the scene investigation, collection of evidence at the scene of the crime and from the pathologist, and transmittal of various articles of evidence to appropriate agencies for ancillary investigations such as photography, fingerprinting, blood typing and ballistic studies. The individual will have to prepare a report dealing with all these aspects of investigation.

It is not usually possible to follow a set pattern in preparing a report;

however, the police investigator in charge of an investigation should specifically include the following information in his report:

1. Date and time of the first call, and the name and address of the person reporting the shooting or fatality

2. Date and time of arrival at the scene of investigation

3. General description of the scene and the names and addresses of the persons present

4. Name and address of the victim with the name and address of the person identifying the victim

5. Details of steps taken to document the findings at the scene

6. Notation of items of evidence collected at the scene with the type of containers used

7. General description of activities of other investigators such as medical examiner, fingerprint investigator, photographer, etc., at the scene of the crime

8. Description of items of evidence collected from the victim's body in the hospital or in the autopsy room

9. Details of disposal of various items of evidence

The police investigator's written record of facts incorporating the above information should also include sworn statements that he may have obtained, photographs made at the scene of the crime and in the autopsy room, photographs of the victim and the items of evidence, diagrams, and receipts establishing the chain of custody of various items that may have been transmitted to other investigators.

The Pathologist's Report

The pathologist's report should consist of a record of the findings of the scene investigation and of the autopsy. The report must include details pertaining to the identification of the victim, documentation of external features and injuries and description of the findings of internal examination, together with conclusions about the cause and manner of death. It is best to document the injuries by photography and by drawings on the body diagram as in Figure 10-1. The information about the gunshot wounds can be conveniently documented on a gunshot wound information chart as illustrated in Figure 10-4. Salient findings of the autopsy can be reflected for quick reference on the front page of the autopsy report as shown in Figure 10-5. It is a good idea to include in the autopsy report a reasonably good-sized, black-and-white identification photograph of the victim. The report file should also include description of the victim's clothing, toxicology report and receipts for materials of evidence given to the police.

The Ballistician's Report

In some instances of crime with a firearm, the firearm examiner may receive a gun, bullets, cartridge cases and clothing for examination. The examiner who makes the ballistic examination must include in his report information related to the source of the evidence examined by him, the date it was received and the method of delivery. The report should also include the date and time of examination of the evidence together with details of the method of examination.

The principal role of a firearms examiner is to help in establishing whether or not a certain firearm was used in the crime. If the weapon suspected to have been used in the crime and the crime bullet and cartridge case are submitted for ballistic examination, all details of the examination of these items should be filled in in appropriate forms used in the laboratory. If a gun is received for examination, the description should include its general condition, type, caliber, make, model, serial number, number of lands and grooves, direction of twist, condition of bore, etc. The description of a bullet should include the degree of damage it shows, its composition, type, make, caliber, weight, number of lands and grooves, direction of twist, etc. If a cartridge or cartridge case is examined, its caliber, make, degree of damage, type of shell, type of crimp should be noted with data on ejector or extractor marks.

After the examination of the evidence bullet and the test fired bullets, the results may be presented in the following simple format.[2]

Report of Positive Results.   A comparison of the evidence bullet and test bullets fired from the suspect weapon was made. The comparison indicated that the evidence bullet was fired from the suspect weapon.

Report of Negative Results.   A comparison of the evidence bullet and test bullets fired from the suspect weapon was made. The comparison indicated that the evidence bullet was not fired from the suspect weapon.

Report of Indeterminate Results.   A comparison of the evidence bullet and test bullets fired from the suspect weapon was made. The comparison did not reveal enough matching individual and accidental markings on the evidence and test bullets to indicate either positively or negatively that the evidence bullet was or was not fired from the suspect weapon.

If for some reason the evidence examined by the firearms examiner leaves his laboratory, he should obtain a signed and dated receipt from the person taking delivery of the evidence. Such a receipt should be preserved with the report on the case.

If the firearms examiner's report is complete and is free from ambiguities, it may be accepted in the court without contest. In fact, in the majority of cases the defense attorney accepts the report of the ballistic expert and his presence in court is not required.

PRESENTATION OF EVIDENCE IN COURT

The police investigator will be required to testify in court in every criminal case that he investigates, because his investigation deals with many facets of the case. On the other hand, the pathologist or the firearms examiner involved in the investigation of medicolegal cases is not summoned to court to testify in all cases. In some jurisdictions, the pathologist is routinely called to present his findings and opinions in the coroner's courts in all cases he investigates. Many higher courts accept the written reports of the pathologist and the firearms examiner, and they do not summon these investigators unless it is thought that questions may be raised about their reports or that their presence would assist in the just disposition of the case. In some instances, they may be asked to give a deposition in order to eliminate the necessity for personal attendance.

The police investigator is usually called as a lay witness or witness of fact, but during the course of testimony he may be required to give opinions on the basis of his experience and thus be used as an expert witness. The ballistician is usually called as an expert because of his specialized task.

Any of these investigators may be required to testify at a preliminary investigation by magistrate, grand jury investigation, coroner's inquest or at trials in criminal courts.

Subpoena

The police officer in charge of the investigation works closely with the prosecuting attorney and usually has information about when the trial is likely to begin. Other investigators usually receive their first notice to appear in court when they are contacted by the police officer, a court official or a lawyer who is in the process of working up the case for trial. The notice may be in the form of a legal subpoena or a telephone call followed later by a subpoena. In some instances, the subpoena may arrive just a few hours prior to the trial, but in most instances, the lawyer for the party who desires the witness's attendance notifies him well in advance of the trial that his presence may be required.

Subpoenas are usually made out for all witnesses to appear in court at the time the trial begins. Frequently, much time is consumed in procedural matters such as picking a jury and settlement of dockets after the court convenes. The police officer is required to be in the court when the trial begins, but it is not always necessary for the pathologist or the ballistician to appear in court at the specified time on the subpoena. It is advisable for him to contact the summoning party to determine the exact time for his appearance in court. In view of the nature of a doctor's work, most attorneys alert the physician some time before his attendance is needed on the day of trial and try to put him on the witness stand promptly when he gets to court.

Preliminaries

Initial Questions.   The witness who receives a subpoena should gather essential information related to the case. He must make sure whether the summoning party is a lawyer for the prosecution or for the defense and whether the case is civil or criminal. The pathologist and the ballistician in particular should find out whether they can give depositions to eliminate the need for personal appearance. If it is necessary to go to court, the witness must locate the court and ascertain when his presence is required.

Pretrial Conference.   A pretrial conference is an ethical procedure. Both the lawyer and the witness should seek to make arrangements for the discussion of the testimony before the witness comes to court. Through such pretrial discussions, the witness gets a clear idea what he will be asked by the attorney calling him. The attorney also is able to advise the witness about the anticipated content of cross-examination. Such discussions give the potential witness an opportunity to find out what records will be required of him. He can point out to the lawyer salient features of the case and advise him about any visual aids such as drawings, photographs and x-rays that may be helpful for his testimony.

Fees.   In some jurisdictions, statutory fees and allowances are laid down for attendance in court. If set fees are nonexistent, it is perfectly in order for the physician and the other independent experts to discuss the question of their fees with the attorney calling or consulting them. The expert witness can expect to be reimbursed for his professional time spent in the preparation of the case, consultations with the attorney and appearance in the court. He should, therefore, keep records of the time that he spends on the case, including travel time. Reimbursement of other investigators, especially police officers, will depend on the terms of their employment.

Preparation of the Case.   Every witness must study the details of the case a few days before he goes to court. It is advisable to review the records again immediately before going to court. The firearms examiner should, in addition, check the comparisons of bullets. All witnesses should make certain that they are conversant with all the information relevant to the case. In some cases, it may be necessary to study the literature on the subject about which they are likely to be cross-examined. This is particularly important if the witness is going to testify as an expert. A witness should not attempt to testify as an expert unless he is satisfied that he is qualified in the subject that is likely to be the focus of questioning.

Materials to be Carried to Court.   The attorney calling the witness will have received copies of the witness's records and other materials before the trial. The witness must carry with him copies of his records so that he can refresh his memory while he is on the witness stand.

The police officer should carry, in addition to his reports, all materials of evidential value. These will include the victim's clothes, weapon, ammunition used in the crime, photographs of relevant evidence, written reports and receipts.

The records of the physician-witness should include the report of the investigation; autopsy report; copy of the death certificate; x-rays; drawings or diagrams; toxicology reports; special reports on swabs or smears, culture studies, serology and blood type studies; and various receipts to prove the chain of custody of the items of evidence. An identification photograph of the decedent's face should also be carried. If the doctor has any other items of physical evidence (e.g., decedent's clothes, bullets) that he is likely to be questioned about, he should carry them with him.

When called to testify, the firearms examiner should take his written reports, all the items of evidence examined by him and any photographs made to illustrate the method of examination or the results. He should also carry a jeweler's loupe or a pocket magnifier.

It is prudent to carry to court the original set of reports and photographs as well as copies of them. Frequently the records and other items of evidence are received in evidence as exhibits. Once they are so received, they become the property of the court and the witness may not get them back. A great many criminal cases are appealed, and there is always a possibility that a new trial may be ordered. One set of records retained by the witness will be invaluable in such circumstances.

Court Attendance

On Arrival at the Court.   Once the time of appearance in court is arranged, the witness should arrive on time with all the necessary records. He should signify to the party who summoned him that he is ready to testify. The sequence of witnesses can vary, but in general the pathologist is called after the preliminary witnesses. The doctor identifies the bullet or bullets that he removed from the body. If the bullet was found at the scene of the crime, the person finding it is called to testify. The police investigator who receives the bullet from the doctor or the person finding it at the scene then identifies the bullet and states that he transmitted the bullet to the firearms examiner. The firearms examiner in turn testifies to the findings of his examination and comparisons of the evidence and test fired bullets.

There may be situations when all the witnesses except the one on the stand are "excluded from the courtroom" prior to their testimony. This is done by the judge upon motion of one of the parties in order that the various witnesses may not hear one another's testimony. The witnesses are also cautioned not to discuss the case with one another while they are waiting to testify. On arrival at the court, therefore, the person called to testify should find out whether the witnesses have been excluded. If they have been excluded, he should signify his arrival to the attorney who called him and then join the other witnesses.

On the Witness Stand. What makes a good witness? According to Tracy, the "attributes of a good medical witness are that he be frank, honest, modest but not timid, have a thorough knowledge of his field of practice, talk to make himself heard, and be able to explain abstruse subjects in language that can be understood by a layman."[4] This statement is perfectly applicable to any other witness.

Following are some simple basic rules that a witness must remember if he is to make a good impression as a witness. These will enhance the effectiveness of his testimony and make his courtroom experience pleasant.

1. Wear neat, conservative clothes.
2. Be relaxed and calm and not frightened or nervous.
3. Do not begin answering until the question is completed.
4. Answer only the question asked and confine yourself to the case on trial.
5. Do not volunteer information uncalled for from the witness stand.
6. Do not answer a question to which an objection has been raised until the judge announces his ruling. If it is overruled, proceed with the answer, but if it is sustained, await another question from the attorney who may rephrase the question or abandon it.
7. Address the answers to the jury.
8. Speak clearly and loudly enough for the jurors to hear.
9. As far as possible use layman's language to explain your testimony.
10. Speak with assurance. Be confident but not overconfident or arrogant. Maintain your composure. Do not lose your temper. Do not argue.
11. Be interested in what is being said. Do not appear bored. "Testifying is similar to a performance on the stage."[3]

12. Do not answer if the question is not understood. Request the attorney to repeat the question or explain it.

13. Be frank, modest and honest. Tell the truth. If you do not know the answer to a question, do not hesitate to say "I do not know." Do not evade a question.

14. Keep the opinions within the realm of reasonableness. Make reasonable deductions. Be fair.

15. If an error has been made in the testimony do not hesitate to correct it.

16. Be pleasant, polite and courteous to the lawyer.

17. Do not underestimate the knowledge of the attorney in the field of your specialty.

After the witness' name is called, he proceeds toward the witness stand. Before he sits in the witness chair, he is sworn in by the clerk of the court. Immediately after this, direct examination commences.

Direct Examination.   This consists of questions put by the attorney who summoned the doctor as a witness. Initial questions are designed to obtain the witness' name, place of residence and occupation. Thereafter, the witness is asked questions bearing upon his qualifications. The medical witness should be prepared to give information about the medical school from which he graduated, his internship and residency training, specialty board certifications, hospital affiliations, research, publications and membershp of medical societies. Other witnesses, likewise, should be ready with an appropriate answer to a question relative to their training, qualifications, experience, affiliations, etc. After establishing the qualifications of the witness, the attorney will ask questions to determine the witness' relation to the case. Once these routine preliminary questions are completed, the attorney will then launch into a more specific line of questioning to bring out the facts and opinions that he considers to be important to his case. This examination will be made without the use of leading questions, that is, questions that suggest their own answers. While answering these questions the witness may consult his records but should refrain from reading from them verbatim. As far as the pathologist is concerned, for instance, the questions usually relate to identification of the decedent, salient autopsy findings and cause of death. The attorney may ask the witness to identify and describe various items of evidence such as reports, photographs, bullets and clothes. If a multipage report is presented for identification, every page of it should be examined before a comment about identification is made.

If a pretrial conference was held, the questions and answers of the direct examination will have been rehearsed and the witness will have no difficulty on the witness stand. Therefore, at least a telephone conference between the attorney and the witness should be arranged prior to the trial.

Cross-Examination.   After the direct examination is completed the opposing attorney will begin questioning the witness. The purpose of this cross-examination is to get the witness to amplify his statements so that the cross-examining attorney can test his memory, and probe the reliability and credibility of his testimony. Many witnesses dread cross-examination, often without justification, because usually no subject may be discussed on cross-examination that has not been opened during the preceding direct examination. Therefore, it is unusual for a witness in a routine medicolegal case to have any problems during cross-examination. The cross-examining attorney may try to impeach the witness in order to diminish the weight of his testimony, by exposing lapses in the investigation or by detecting discrepancies in the statements made during the direct examination and the cross-examination. So, if the investigation of the case has been proper and the witness has presented forthright factual testimony on direct examination, he need not fear a vigorous cross-examination.

After the cross-examination is completed, there may be *redirect examination.* On redirect examination the lawyer who calls the witness usually tries to give him an opportunity to explain his answers given during cross-examination. If any new issues are introduced during redirect examination, the opposing attorney may pursue a *recross-examination.* Details of these examinations are well discussed by Beeman.[1]

After both parties have completed their direct and cross-examinations and all the evidence that may be desired from the witness has been introduced, he will be excused from the witness stand. At this stage the witness should ask the judge to be excused from the case totally. Such a request is usually granted and the witness is then free to leave the court.

In summary, it must be reemphasized that if the witness makes prior arrangements with the attorney about the precise time of appearance in the court, he is not likely to spend unnecessary time there. Further, if he prepares the case properly and confers with the calling attorney before testifying, his task in court will be rendered easy. Finally, most trial lawyers conduct themselves as gentlemen; hence, a truthful, prepared witness should have nothing to fear in the court.

REFERENCES

1. Beeman, J.: The Pathologist As a Witness. Mundelein, (Ill.), Callaghan, 1964.
2. Hatcher, J. S., Jury, F. J. and Weller, J.: Firearms Investigation, Identification and Evidence. Harrisburg, Stackpole, 1957.
3. Liebenson, H.: You, the Medical Witness. Mundelein, (Ill.), Callaghan, 1961.
4. Tracy, J. E.: The Doctor As a Witness. Philadelphia, W. B. Saunders, 1957.

Index

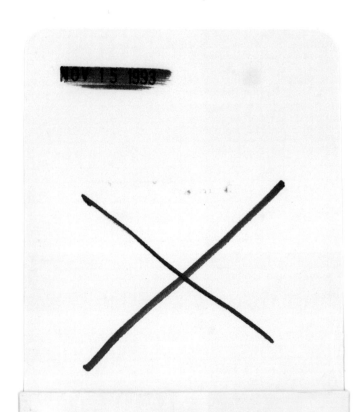